Slip Sliding Away

TURNING BACK THE CLOCK ON YOUR VAGINA

By Lauren Streicher, MD

This book is not intended
to replace medical advice and
should be used to supplement, not replace,
care by your personal health care clinician.
The publisher and author disclaim liability
for any medical outcomes that may occur as
a result of applying methods suggested or
discussed in this book.

About Lauren Streicher, MD, FACOG, NCMP

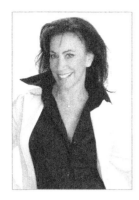 DR. LAUREN STREICHER is a best-selling author, a Clinical Professor of Obstetrics and Gynecology at Northwestern University's Medical School, the Feinberg School of Medicine, a Certified Menopause Practitioner of The North American Menopause Society, and the medical director of the Northwestern Medicine Center for Menopause and the Northwestern Medicine Center for Sexual Medicine. In addition to her consumer books and articles, she has authored multiple scientific publications. Dr. Streicher is routinely interviewed as a reliable, accurate source for national publications such as The New York Times, Newsweek, the Associated Press and dozens of magazines. She writes a monthly column for Prevention Magazine. She was the 2019 recipient of the North American Menopause Society Media Award.

Dr. Streicher is the Medical Correspondent for Chicago's top rated news program, the WGN Morning News, and has multiple appearances on The Today Show, Good Morning America, The Oprah Winfrey Show, CNN, NPR, Dr. Radio, Nightline, The Dr. Oz Show, Fox and Friends, The Steve Harvey Show, CBS this Morning, ABC News Now, NBC Nightly news, 20/20, and World News Tonight.

She lives in Chicago with her writer-producer husband, Jason Brett, and their dog KJ. They have four grown daughters.

Other books by Dr. Streicher:
The Essential Guide to Hysterectomy
1st edition M. Evans & Company
2nd edition M. Evans & Company

Sex Rx: Hormones Health and Your Best Sex Ever
Harper Collins (Originally released as *Love Sex Again*)

Contents

CONTENTS

Chapter 14

RESOURCES AND TERMINOLOGY
Books, websites and further information.

Acknowledgments

*The saga of Francey's
journey through menopause continues!*

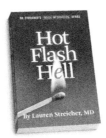

DR. STREICHER'S INSIDE INFORMATION:
Hot Flash Hell *(July 2021)*

DR. STREICHER'S INSIDE INFORMATION:
**Dating After 40—
Making It Awesome Instead of Awful** *(October 2021)*

DR. STREICHER'S INSIDE INFORMATION:
Cancer and Sex *(January 2022)*

DR. STREICHER'S INSIDE INFORMATION:
Finding Your Menopause Mojo *(April 2022)*

DR. STREICHER'S INSIDE INFORMATION:
Incontinence—Say "No!" to Diapers *(August 2022)*

DR. STREICHER'S INSIDE INFORMATION:
Post-40 Skin, Hair, and Nails *(November 2022)*

To Jason- the love of my life

In loving memory of my parents,
Lyle Bass Streicher and Dr. Daniel Streicher

Introduction

IF EVERY MAN woke up on his 50th birthday and started having all-day, all-night hot flashes, couldn't think, and couldn't function, if his bones started to deteriorate at an alarming rate, if his risk for heart disease dramatically increased, if his penis shrunk to the size of a breakfast sausage, and if he were incapable of any sexual activity, he would not be told, "This is a normal part of aging." He would be given solutions. Lots of them.

Yet the eighty percent of menopausal women who experience symptoms that impede their ability to think, sleep, work, and function sexually are expected to put up with hot flashes, vaginal dryness, weight gain, and insomnia. For most women, this occurs when they are at the prime of their professional and personal lives, but these changes can happen even earlier if someone enters menopause as a result of chemotherapy, radiation, medication, or surgery.

In addition, we now know that hot flashes result in an inflammatory response that accelerates vascular changes that lead to heart disease or stroke.

So, it's not just quality of life—it is also length of life.

Many women assume that menopause is temporary, and once the hot flashes go away, menopause is over. But menopause is never over. You do not go through menopause. You enter menopause. Even if you are no longer having hot flashes, the impact of no longer producing estrogen is forever.

It doesn't have to be this way. There are safe, effective treatments that most women are not offered and arc not aware of that will protect your bones, your bladder, your brain, your heart, your sex life, and your sanity.

I am solution-driven, and my mission is to address this enormous, unmet need by giving women good information so they can make good choices.

That's why I decided to write my Inside Information Series as a collection of guides that will enable you to navigate the individual issues you are trying to fix. You may end up reading the whole series, or just one book.

Slip Sliding Away: Turning Back the Clock on Your Vagina is specifically about all the hormonal and non-hormonal options to alleviate the vulvar, vaginal, and urinary symptoms that result from a lack of estrogen.

So, to that end, meet Francey.

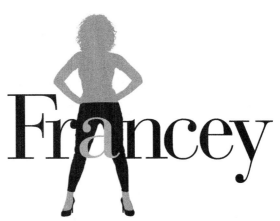

SHE IS 49 YEARS old and newly single, with three grown children. Despite spending her twenties and thirties loving sex and having a lot of it, it's been a decade since she has even thought about her genitals. With the kids out of the house, Francey is ready for a fresh start, which includes bringing her vagina out of retirement. But, like millions of peri-menopausal and menopausal women across the country, Francey's vagina appears to be all dried up. Slip Sliding Away is the story of Francey's vagina—and how she finds lubrication.

Slip Sliding Away

TURNING BACK THE CLOCK ON YOUR VAGINA

A GYNECOLOGIST'S GUIDE
TO ELIMINATING
POST-MENOPAUSE
DRYNESS AND PAIN

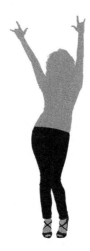

> AFTER A THREE-YEAR sexual hiatus, thanks to a series of first dates with nothing but narcissistic jerks, Francey, 49, finally connects with Adam, 48, who is smart, interesting, and refreshingly willing to date age-appropriate women. Bonus: He is also a fabulous kisser who appreciates the value of meticulous dental hygiene. In preparation for a romantic evening, Francey splurges on a very expensive bra to enhance her not-as-perky-as-they-used-to-be breasts and stages her apartment with plenty of candlelight (after all, time and three kids have not been kind to her thighs and tush). Not to worry: Within five minutes of Adam's arrival, the bra is off, and there is no indication that her less-than-model-like body is a problem.

But there is another problem: Despite Francey's excitement, Adam's penis encounters the equivalent of the Sahara desert.

Adam, being a guy (who has been dating age-appropriate women), dashes to the kitchen, checks the cabinets, then returns with the coconut oil Francey purchased a few months ago during a baking frenzy. He expertly slathers the oil all over his penis and the opening to Francey's vagina. Success!

1

WHOSE VAGINA IS THIS
AND WHY IS IT ON MY BODY?

PRIOR TO 1998, men who were unable to maintain an erection were said to suffer from impotency. Think about it. It's bad enough to have a penis that won't cooperate, but then to have a diagnosis that implies you are also weak, incompetent, and powerless is too much to expect any man to deal with. A guy who was impotent didn't just have a medical problem. He was a personal failure. No way was he going to make an appointment to discuss his impotency with his medical doctor. The poor guys had to suffer in silence.

In 1998, the impotent man disappeared. Enter the man with ED. The man with ED was handsome, successful, and sexy. The man with ED felt so powerful that Senator Bob Dole, a presidential candidate, went on national TV to proudly talk about his newly functional penis.

So who propagated the term "erectile dysfunction"? The people who had a lot to gain from men admitting they had a problem. I think you know where I'm going. It was the inventors of Viagra™ who launched one of the most brilliant marketing successes of the 20th century. Pfizer launched Viagra™ and at the same time launched a marketing campaign that redefined impotency as erectile dysfunction. The condition was not only normalized, but it also gave men the language (ED!) to talk to their doctor about it so they could comfortably ask for a prescription.

Why am I even bringing this up? Well, for every man who suffers from erectile dysfunction, there is a woman who suffers from vaginal atrophy. Women with vaginal atrophy resulting from the hormonal changes that occur during the transition to menopause have vaginal walls that are so thin and dry that intercourse is either excruciatingly painful or impossible.

But, like men who are impotent, no women (even if they are familiar with the term) want to have vaginal atrophy! Talk about a buzz kill. "Honey, my vagina is atrophied. I can't have sex tonight. Or ever."

Right now, in the United States, there are over fifty million women who are no longer producing estrogen, and another few million are peri-menopausal. Despite the fact that sixty percent of these women avoid or have abandoned sex as a result of dry, thin vaginal walls, only seven percent of women are treated despite the availability of safe and effective options to make sex pleasurable and, in many cases, possible.

For the millions of women who have vaginal (and vulvar) atrophy and have lost the ability to have pleasurable, slippery sex, I came up with a solution—my version of ED for women.

Instead of using the term "vaginal atrophy" (which no one knows, can remember, or wants to say), when I wrote Sex Rx, I attempted to introduce a new term: "genital dryness," or GD. Just as guys found it easier to say they had ED than to announce they were impotent, I thought women would find it much easier to say they had GD. I know—it's brilliant. But it didn't catch on. So I suggest women now simply say they have vaginal dryness. But if GD ever does catch on, you heard it here first.

I want to emphasize that vaginal atrophy is not the only genital consequence of menopause. Even if sex is not desired, the hormonal changes that occur also cause nonsexual genital issues such as irritation, burning, and urinary symptoms.

Genitourinary syndrome of menopause, or GSM, is the medical terminology that was introduced in 2013. It acknowledges that a lack of estrogen affects not only the vagina, but also the vulva (external genitalia) and the urinary tract.

Physical changes that occur as a result of genitourinary syndrome of menopause

- Thin, dry vaginal and vulvar tissue
- Decreased elasticity
- Shortening and shrinkage of the labia
- Pallor (pink tissue becomes pale tissue)
- Loss of vaginal rugae (the accordion-like folds in the vagina that allow for expansion during intercourse)
- Vaginal mucosal fragility (tissue that bleeds easily)
- Elevation of vaginal pH and alteration of the vaginal microbiome (the healthy bacteria that populate the vagina)
- Funneling of the urethra (the urethra pokes out instead of lying flat)

Symptoms that occur because of genitourinary syndrome of menopause

- Decreased lubrication with sexual activity
- Pain with sexual activity and intercourse
- Vulvar and vaginal itching, burning, and irritation
- Urinary frequency
- Urinary urgency (that constant "gotta go" feeling)
- Recurrent urinary tract infections

No surprise, the consequences of these changes go way beyond the ability to have pain-free, enjoyable sex. Multiple studies show that women with GSM also experience loss of libido, difficulty having an orgasm, avoidance of intimacy, and interference with sexual spontaneity.

My clinical experience mirrors what is in the medical literature. Ask pretty much any woman who has experienced the pain of "sandpaper sex" and she will tell you that her "solution" to prevent repeat agony is to go into avoidance mode. Aside from the obvious loss of physical pleasure, it stands to reason that cleaning out the linen closet at 10 p.m. instead of a rendezvous in the bedroom is likely to have a negative impact on one's relationship and quality of life.

Women who are brave enough to ask their doctor get little or no information and no solutions beyond "try a lubricant."

Lack of estrogen is not just about the changes that occur in the vagina. Atrophy in the urinary tract results in a number of tissue alterations including inflammation of the urethra. Woman who get up three times a night to pee, and are constantly dealing with a sudden, irresistible urge to void, usually have no idea that their urinary urgency is a direct result of menopause.

At its extreme, urge incontinence, the bladder muscles contract when they should not, resulting in involuntary loss of urine. The woman with urge incontinence is fine until she puts her key in the door. If she is lucky, the door will open, she won't drop her packages, and she will make it to the toilet and get her pants down within the next four seconds. It is no surprise that falls occur twice as often in women with urge incontinence than those without bladder symptoms. And don't get me started on the multi-million dollar diaper industry that has normalized this treatable condition that affects up to fifty percent of post menopause women.

> ❯ *TWO DAYS AFTER her date with Adam, Francey woke up with that constant "gotta go" feeling. Then came the knife like pain with urination followed by the terrifying sight of pee the color of cranberry juice. Having experienced this before, Francey immediately knew the diagnosis: the dreaded urinary tract infection...*

The only thing more miserable than a urinary tract infection is when it happens again, and again, and again. Those recurrent urinary tract infections, occur when bacteria (usually E.coli) that normally populates the gastrointestinal tract makes its way to the urethra and then travels up to the bladder. E.coli proliferate and are more likely take up residence in the urethra when healthy vaginal lactobacilli get wiped out—a scenario, which can occur in young women but is even more common post menopause as a consequence of elevated pH due to lack of estrogen. In addition, the female urethra is a much shorter (and more traveled) road than a male urethra which is why women are the ones that suffer. It is also why woman who have a short distance between the anus and urethra are more likely to get infected than other women.

Hence, post menopause women are prime candidates for recurrent urinary tract infection (UTI) which is defined as more than two infections in six months or more than three infections in one year.

While plenty of women who haven't been near a penis in years get recurrent bladder infections, sexual intercourse (especially with a new partner) dramatically increases the risk. Intimate contact (no matter how many showers you take, how often you pee and how well you wipe) facilitates the journey of E.coli from the rectum to the urethra. And while condoms and spermicide decrease the chance of an STI, sadly, being responsible about protection is no defense against a UTI. In some cases, a spermicide increases the risk.

New Partner + Menopause + Lots of Sex = Perfect UTI Storm

Women who get recurrent urinary tract infections get recurrent antibiotics which in turn leads to recurrent yeast infections. This is especially problematic since a 2021 study showed that in more than 76% of cases, antibiotics to treat a bladder infection are prescribed for more days than are needed to wipe out the infection, Even worse, some women end up getting a cystoscopy (a surgical procedure performed by a urologist) to look inside the bladder.

If all of this sounds familiar, (vaginal dryness, painful sex, irritation, burning and recurrent bladder infections) you are in the right place.

These are fixable problems, and far too many women needlessly suffer. But the solutions are not one-size-fits-all any more than one speculum fits all! The women who have only mild GSM may be fine with the right lubricant; other women may need to turn to a prescription remedy. Some women will also need to work with a pelvic floor physical therapist. It's not always enough to treat the tissue. The underlying muscles have been in "keep out!" mode so long that they may also need some help.

What follows is your road map to restore your ability to have pain-free intercourse and also eliminate other bothersome symptoms of GSM. Slip Sliding Away is very specific. It does not cover problems with libido, difficulty having orgasms, or painful intercourse from causes other than menopause. It does not cover the psychosocial aspects of human sexuality. It does not cover other menopause issues such as hot flashes, bone health, and cognitive function. Those topics will be covered in other Inside Information Guides.

So arm yourself with information and soon you will be slip sliding away! ▼

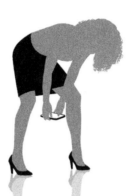

> ONCE THE ANTIBIOTICS kick in and she is no longer peeing (and screaming) every ten minutes, Francey decides it's time to investigate what is going on. Admittedly, she hadn't paid a lot of attention to her vagina for at least ten years, but something is definitely not OK. She tries to take a crotch selfie, but it is just a big blur. Next, she perches on the edge of the bathtub with her feet propped on the toilet and uses a mirror and a flashlight to get a slightly better view. Her labia look kind of red and actually a lot shorter than she remembers. Panic sets in: Are her labia disappearing?

2

WHAT'S UP DOWN THERE?

MEN HAVE ALWAYS had the clear advantage of being able to inspect their genitals with very little effort on their part. Women's genitals are not quite as accessible, resulting in a lot more uncertainty about what's normal and what's not. Too often women are told: "It's nasty down there!" "Don't look!" "Don't touch!" For many women, the first time they take a really good look (or attempt to take a good look) is when they think something is wrong. And ninety percent of the time, when a woman is referring to her vagina, as in "I have a rash on my vagina," she is referring to her vulva.

The vulva is defined as female external genitalia and includes the mons pubis (including pubic hair), labia, clitoris, vestibule, hymen, and perineum. Basically, the vulva includes all the parts you can see without any special instruments. The vagina is inside, and unless you own a speculum, it's not something you can see on your own.

So here is a list of the parts, what they look like pre-menopause, and the physical changes that can occur because of age and menopause. Although the average age to stop menstruating is 52, vaginal changes can begin as early as age 40, long before you officially donate your tampons to your daughter. And if you skipped the part in

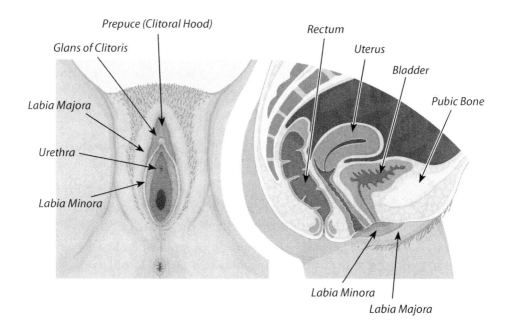

chapter 1 about genitourinary syndrome of menopause, you need to go back and read it now. Sorry.

Also, in this guide I am not going to get into the nitty-gritty of medical conditions that cause problems (outside of menopause) but suffice it to say that anything that is painful, itchy, discolored, or rashy—along with any new lumps, bumps, or blisters—needs to be checked out by a doctor.

PUBIC HAIR

The distribution of hair as well as its color and coarseness are genetically determined, with a wide range of what is considered normal. Pubic hair actually has a biologic function. Before central heating, pubic hair kept the genitals warm. The obvious advantage of warm genitals is that people would be more likely to take their clothes off, and men would be more likely to maintain an erection. From an evolutionary point of view, the other function of pubic hair is to draw attention to the genitals. (Evidently it is not just modern men who seem to need a map to ensure they are heading in the right direction). Pubic hair also decreases friction during intercourse –I've seen some pretty nasty "rug burn" from rubbing while bare.

What I see is often not a reflection of what is really going on, because changing trends in hairstyles are not limited to the hair on your head. As a gynecologist, I get a firsthand view of what's fashionable. Today less is more, and many women I see alter their pubic hair in some way, whether it's just a trim or complete removal. Along with the "less is more" trend comes the ability to clearly see what things look like, and many women often spend an inordinate amount of time and energy worrying about the appearance of their external genitalia. Being self-critical is evidently not limited to worrying about one's butt and thighs.

Pre-menopause:

Left untouched, the pubic hair of most young women ranges in its thickness, texture, and abundance. Some women have a sprinkling of scant, fine hair, while others have coarse, curly hair that not only covers the mons but also creeps up the abdomen and down the thighs.

Post-menopause:

Hormones influence hair growth, so it makes sense that as women age and hormones decline, pubic hair thins out. It is not unusual for a woman in her seventies or eighties to have very little to no pubic hair. And, yes, just like the hair on your head, genital hair can go gray, but strangely enough, not always both at the same time. Although some women dye their grays, I don't recommend it. I have seen a number of dyeing disasters, including one really nasty clitoral burn that landed my patient in the hospital.

VULVAR SKIN

Pre-menopause:

The skin on the vulva should appear similar to the skin everywhere else on your body.

Post-menopause:

It is not unusual for vulvar skin to become pale and thin. Of course, any inflammation, rashes, new growths, discolorations, ulcerations, bleeding, burning or very itchy areas should be checked out by your doctor.

CLITORIS

Although it just seems like a little pea, the clitoris is a bundle of nerves that dives into the body and can be up to four inches long. In other words, what you see is just the tip of the iceberg. It is still considered to be part of the external genitalia even though the internal segment, which extends to just under the pubic bone, is longer than the external component. The part that is visible is called the glans. The glans is often partially or completely covered by the prepuce, which looks like a little hood. The corpus cavernosa of the clitoris is comprised of erectile tissue and run along the sides the vaginal opening.

STRUCTURE OF THE CLITORIS

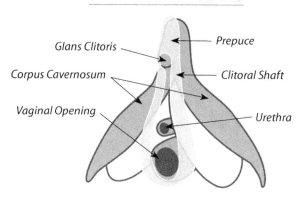

Pre-menopause:

The clitoris should be rosy pink and roughly the size of a Q-tip. Normally the hood easily slides off the clitoris to expose part or all of the glans.

Post-menopause:

There is usually not a dramatic change later in life, but it is not unusual for the glans to appear a little paler and smaller. If the clitoris is buried, it may be a result of atrophic changes, but it may also mean there is a vulvar condition, such as lichen sclerosus. And, yes, orgasm is still possible even if the clitoris is not visible. Phew!

URETHRA

The urethra is the tube that carries urine from the bladder to the outside. The urethra is about an inch long, but you only see the opening, known as the meatus, where the urine comes out. It is positioned inside the vestibule, below the clitoris.

Pre-menopause:

It's not always easy to see, but if you are able to, it is a little opening that protrudes only slightly from the surrounding tissue.

Post-menopause:

The urethral opening can suddenly be a lot more prominent and easily visible just by parting the labia minora. This anatomic change is known as urethral funneling and is a good indication that the vaginal and vestibular tissue are dry and thin.

LABIA MAJORA

The labia majora refer to the "large" or outer lips that surround the vagina. The labia majora are folds that include the skin and fatty tissue that start at the mons pubis and extend to about an inch above the anus.

Pre-menopause:

The labia majora tend to be plump and full, but body type has a huge impact on appearance, and there is a wide range of normal.

Post-menopause:

Unlike your hips, the labia majora tend to get thinner post-menopause. The skin is also dryer. The labia majora often appear to be bigger, but that is actually an optical illusion. It's the labial fat that has diminished, making the labia majora seem more pendulous.

LABIA MINORA

The labia minora are the lips that surround the "mouth" of the vagina. Unlike the labia majora, the labia minora have no fatty tissue and are very thin. The labia minora start at the clitoral hood and, in most cases, end right below the vaginal opening. In many women, the labia minora only extend partway down the opening of the vagina. There are as many shapes and lengths of labia minora as there are snowflakes.

Pre-menopause:

The average labia minora measures less than three centimeters from base to tip, but obviously there's a huge range of what is considered normal.

Post-menopause:

As women age and estrogen levels decline, the color tends to fade. In addition, the labia minora become shorter and thinner, and, in some cases, flatten out and can even disappear. This process, known as agglutination, starts at the bottom and can progress all the way to the top.

VESTIBULE

The vestibule refers to the area immediately outside of the vagina, starting from the hymen (or what's left of it!)

and ending with the labia minora. The vestibule has a rich nerve supply, which is why it is the area that is most likely to be painful, uncomfortable, or itchy if there is an infection or dryness. When most women refer to their vagina, they are usually referring to the vestibule. The vestibule should be pain-free when touched.

Pre-menopause:
The vestibule is usually rosy pink and pain free.

Post-menopause:
A pale vestibule, which can turn practically white, is a consequence of decreased blood supply. Sometimes the tissue is so dry and inflamed that there are bright red, painful patches. This area can be a major source of pain.

INTROITUS

The introitus is the port of entry into the vagina. and is marked by the hymen in virgins, or hymeneal remnants in someone who has had intercourse.

Pre-menopause:
In a young woman, the introitus is often not visible without separating the labia minora with fingers. A "relaxed" hymen or introitus refers to a vaginal opening which appears gaping or stretched out. This is typically seen in women who have had vaginal deliveries. In general, a gaping introitus is not a cause of pain or sexual dysfunction.

Post-menopause:
In a post-menopausal woman, the appearance is even more variable, depending on if she delivered vaginally, how much relaxation is present, the degree of atrophy, and if she has remained sexually active. In women with severe atrophy, the introitus shrinks.

VAGINA

The vagina is an internal, tubelike organ that begins at

the hymen and ends at the cervix. The length of a normal vagina is not only highly variable and dependent on sexual arousal, but it also varies as a result of childbirth, body habitus, and sexual practices. Before Botox, one look at a woman's face told her age. Now one has to rely on the appearance of the inside of her vagina to know if she is in the over-fifty club. The vagina doesn't lie.

There are a number of features of the vagina that indicate vaginal health and hormonal status.

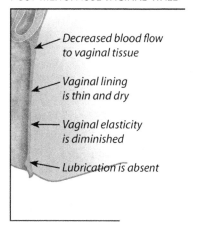

PRE-MENOPAUSE VAGINAL WALL   POST-MENOPAUSE VAGINAL WALL

Good blood flow to vaginal tissue

Vaginal lining is thick and moist

Vaginal walls are elastic

Lubrication is present

Decreased blood flow to vaginal tissue

Vaginal lining is thin and dry

Vaginal elasticity is diminished

Lubrication is absent

Pre-menopause:
- Color: The color should be a rich, deep pink.
- Rugae: These are the accordion-like folds of the wall of the vagina that allow for maximum elasticity and stretchability.
- Vaginal wall thickness: A normal vaginal wall is about three to four millimeters thick.
- Lubrication: The walls of the vagina should appear moist and glistening.

Post-menopause:
- Color: The pink often fades to practically white.

- Rugae: Those accordion-like folds of the wall of the vagina become flatter and often disappear. Along with the disappearance of the rugae comes the disappearance of stretchability and elasticity.
- Vaginal wall thickness: With age and lack of estrogen, the walls become thinner. The loss of the top layer, the epithelium, is the biggest problem because this is the part of the vaginal wall that is primarily responsible for lubrication. In cases of severe atrophy, the vaginal wall bleeds easily.
- Lubrication: It's history.

If you put the vaginal wall under a microscope (I know, most women do not generally put their vaginal wall under a microscope), the changes are really obvious. The all-important top layer (containing the epithelial cells) is critical when it comes to lubrication and elasticity. And in seventy percent of post-menopause vaginal walls, if left untreated, the epithelial layer is pretty much nonexistent. The goal of many treatments described in subsequent chapters is to restore the epithelial layer to its pre-menopause state.

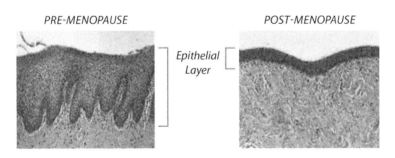

PRE-MENOPAUSE   POST-MENOPAUSE

Epithelial
Layer

So now that you have seen my view from the other side of the stirrups, it's time to get out a mirror (preferably with magnification), a decent light, and take a tour of your own vulva. ▼

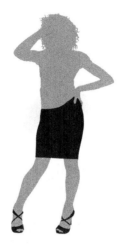

> *AND THEN CAME the irritating itch. Before long, Francey finds herself absentmindedly scratching the opening to her vagina while she watches the news or scrolls through Facebook posts. During a romantic dinner with Adam, she even has to leave the table (during dessert!) to scratch her itch. She recently started using a new feminine wash, and it dawns on her that despite her genitals now smelling like an English garden, it may be the culprit. Sure enough, when she stops using it, the irritation and redness go away. Everything is great until two weeks later, when Francey once again develops an itchy, red vulva. Of course, she suspects gonorrhea or syphilis, but her gynecologist reassures her that it's only a yeast infection, possibly from using coconut oil as a lubricant. After popping a Diflucan™ and avoiding sexual activity for a few days, all is right again.*

3

A TRIP DOWN THE FEMININE HYGIENE AISLE

EVERY GYNECOLOGIST KNOWS that "feminine hygiene" is big business- ("feminine" of course being the acceptable marketing euphemism for "vaginal"), but it was surprising even to me to learn just how big. A search of "feminine hygiene" products on Amazon.com yields over two thousand results. In fairness, that incudes menstrual products such as pads, tampons and cups, but a query using the phrase "feminine odor" still results in well over one thousand options for odor-reducing products to be used either externally (on the vulva) or internally (in the vagina).

In contrast, a "male hygiene" search yielded only a handful of products for "odor control," including "Topp Cock-Hygiene™ for Man Parts" and my personal favorite, "Fresh Balls™." "Defunk your junk" is its actual ad. I couldn't make this stuff up.

Are vaginas so smelly that there need to be thousands of products and a billion-dollar industry to eliminate the stench? As a gynecologist, and a woman, I find the implication that a woman's genitals are in constant need of cleaning and perfuming so that they are not offensive, offensive.

The phrase "feminine hygiene" was coined in 1873 as a response to the Comstock Act, which made it a federal crime to distribute contraception-related materials. In response, the birth control industry coined the term "feminine hygiene" to advertise and sell over-the-counter contraception. The term was never intended to refer to vaginal odor, cleansing the genitalia, or, god forbid, using genital perfume.

When Your Vagina Is in a pHunk

I also see many women worried about perceived vaginal odor who have no problem but have been conditioned (by the feminine hygiene industry and sometimes a well-meaning mother or clueless partner) to believe that all vaginas are naturally offensive and smelly even when all is well.

Vaginal shaming is not a new phenomenon. In the 1950s, women were advised to douche with Lysol to prevent odor and avoid losing their husbands.

However, if there is a foul, fishy odor despite a daily shower and basic hygiene, the most likely culprit is an alteration of pH, which refers to the vagina's acidity level.

A healthy vaginal microbiome is predominantly populated with beneficial bacteria, the lactobacilli, which produce lactic acid and keep vaginal pH in a low, healthy range. A low pH keeps good bacteria (lactobacilli) in balance and decreases the opportunities for bad bacteria (Gardnerella) to grow. Women of reproductive age (after puberty and before menopause) normally maintain a healthy vaginal pH between 3.5 and 5 on a scale of 0 to 14. Post-menopause, the pH rises and there is an alteration in the microbiome, which in turn increases the risk of infection.

If Gardnerella predominates, the result is a funky odor. At its extreme, the result of too much bad bacteria is bacterial vaginosis (BV). BV, not yeast, is the most common cause of abnormal vaginal discharge, accounting for forty

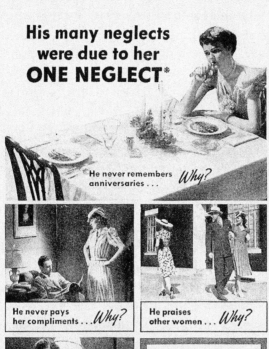

His many neglects were due to her ONE NEGLECT*

He never remembers anniversaries ... *Why?*

He never pays her compliments ... *Why?*

He praises other women ... *Why?*

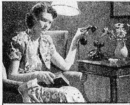

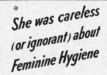

He's often "kept downtown".. *Why?*

* She was careless (or ignorant) about Feminine Hygiene

This one neglect may be the real cause of many divorces...Use "LYSOL" for Feminine Hygiene.

Let "Lysol" help YOU to avoid this ONE NEGLECT!

IF THERE is any doubt in *your* mind about this important subject of feminine hygiene, ask your doctor about "Lysol". Let him tell you why, for a full half-century, "Lysol" has earned the confidence of so many doctors, nurses, hospitals ... *and wives.* Probably no other product is so widely used for this purpose. Three sizes of "Lysol" are sold at all drug stores.

Lysol Disinfectant

1889—1939
50th ANNIVERSARY

What Every Woman Should Know
SEND COUPON FOR "LYSOL" BOOKLET
LEHN & FINK PRODUCTS CORP.
Dept. M.P.-908, Bloomfield, N. J., U. S. A.
Send me free booklet "Lysol vs. Germs" which tells the many uses of "Lysol".

Name

Address
Copyright 1939 by Lehn & Fink Products Corp.

Vaginal shaming is not a new phenomenon. In the 1950s, women were advised to douche with Lysol to prevent odor and avoid losing their husbands.

to fifty percent of cases. But it's not just about an irritating discharge. Women with BV are at risk for many more serious medical conditions, including an increased tendency to acquire sexually transmitted infections such as gonorrhea and chlamydia.

When things seem to be awry, it's understandably tempting to dash to the store and get a basketful of products that promise to keep your vagina smelling like a flower shop. But before you make that expensive run, you need to know which products might actually help and which ones may make matters worse.

Products to Prevent Odor

External washes and wipes are promoted as essential to keep your vulva clean and odor-free. That's fine in concept, but most of these products are not only unnecessary but also potentially irritating to delicate vulvar skin. Many of these washes and wipes are loaded with preservatives, perfumes, and additives that cause inflammation. Most promise to keep your vulva "pH-balanced" as a strategy to prevent vaginal odor from starting. But if you think about it, that approach is biologically impossible.

Using a pH-balanced vulvar wash to balance vaginal pH (and control odor) is akin to washing your face in order to prevent bad breath.

Products to Eliminate or Cover Up Odor

Vulvar and vaginal deodorant sprays, powders, panty liners, and washes are essentially perfume to camouflage genital odor. Even if you want your vagina to smell like a Tahitian sunset, tropical rain, or a Mandarin blossom, keep in mind that, like vulvar washes, these products are loaded with preservatives and chemicals that can cause irritation, burning, and redness.

Other Vulvar Irritants to Avoid

Vulvar washes and deodorants are not the only products that can cause irritation and inflammation. A general rule of thumb is that if you can't pronounce the ingredients in an over-the-counter product, you probably should not be putting it on your vulva. Although many women get away with using these products without damaging and irritating the tissue, most post-menopause vaginas and vulvas needs extra TLC.

Tips to Avoid Irritation to Vulvar Tissue

- Do not use any douches, perfumes, antiperspirants, deodorants, or creams on your vulva.
- Vagisil™ and other over-the-counter vaginal itch medications that contain benzocaine, a topical anesthetic/numbing medication, are particularly toxic and can cause severe skin problems.
- Avoid bubble baths.
- No scented toilet paper!
- For women who wear a protective pad because of urine leakage, be sure to use only fragrance-free, unscented ones.
- Change pads often to minimize moisture and irritation (urine is really irritating to vulvar tissues).
- Wash underwear and clothing in fragrance-free, dye-free laundry detergent with an extra rinse cycle.
- Forget the fabric softener when washing your underwear.
- And speaking of underwear: Leave it off when you go to bed.

Don't be reassured by phrases such as "gynecologist tested" and "doctor recommended," which are meaningless and may simply mean a gynecologist (employed by the company) sprayed it on a few patients and nothing bad happened.

Patient testimonials of efficacy are also not credible. Products that have been scientifically tested will usually cite clinically relevant medical publications on their website.

The Care and Cleaning of Your Vulva and Vagina

So now that I have given you a milelong list of things not to do, what should you do to stay clean and fresh? It's simple.

There is never a need to clean your genitals internally. Your vagina is self-cleaning.

There is no need to clean your genitals externally using anything other than simple soap and water. Stick to fragrance-free, neutral cleansers—examples include Basis™ bar soap, Vanicream™ bar soap, Cetaphil™ bar soap, Cetaphil™ liquid cleanser, and Aquanil™ cleanser. If you use a vulvar wipe, choose one that is unscented, hypoallergenic, and chemical- and preservative-free, which will most likely be found in the baby aisle. Water Wipes™ (available at most drugstores) contain 99.9% water and a drop of grapefruit seed extract and is a safe option.

If you are having vulvar issues, your best bet is to stop using soap. Just clean your vulva with water. I promise you, there will be no odor. Avoid toilet paper altogether, and spray lukewarm water on the vulva using a sports water bottle or perineum care bottle.

If you have discomfort or burning during urination, pour or spray lukewarm water over the vulva WHILE you are urinating. Gently pat dry.

When it comes to lubricant—the mother of vulvar irritants—check out chapter 4 for a list of products that are not irritating.

Bottom line: If you have an offensive odor, get rid of it—don't mask it! In some cases, the pH is "off " just enough to cause an odor without your having full-blown bacterial vaginosis. A reasonable first step if things smell a little funky is to use RePhresh™, an over-the-counter gel that will balance the pH and give your own lactobacilli a fighting chance to get things in order.

Although douching is an incredibly tempting "quick fix," it will freshen things up only for about ten seconds and then inevitably make things worse. Not only can douching elevate the pH, but it also dehydrates tissues and washes away whatever lactobacilli you have. Scented douches can irritate things even more. In addition, douching is associated with an increase in ectopic pregnancies, pelvic inflammatory disease, and subsequent infertility. That's not relevant to the over-fifty crowd, but it is information you need to tell your daughters!

What About Those Recurrent Bladder Infections?

Drugstore aisles and online marketplaces are loaded with products that claim to "cleanse your urinary tract," "flush impurities," "support bladder health," and, no surprise, "prevent urinary tract infections." Despite what your mother, your hairdresser, your favorite magazine, or even your actual doctor has told you, scientific studies have not shown that any of those supplements, or any of the following interventions, reduce the chance of recurrent infections.

1. Peeing immediately before and immediately after intercourse (no more leaping out of bed!)
2. Frequent urination (you have better things to do)
3. Wiping patterns (front to back, back to front—I know, but really, it makes no difference!)
4. Hot tubs (enjoy, but forget the bubbles)

5. Pantyhose (phew)
6. Cranberry juice (delicious but not helpful)

So Give Me Some Good News

If a UTI is properly treated (and a woman has an anatomically normal urinary tract), even frequently recurrent UTIs will not lead to long-term health problems such as kidney disease. And, yes, there are action steps that do work to reduce or eliminate recurrence.

1. Drink more water! In a 2020 study, young women with recurrent UTIs who increased their daily intake of water to two to three liters reduced their recurrence rate by fifty percent! This does not work once you have a UTI; increasing your water intake must be done on a regular basis to flush out sticky bacteria and prevent infection. It stands to reason that this would help the post-menopause crowd as well.

2. Eliminate the use of products with spermicide, such as condoms and diaphragms. Use a condom without spermicide for STI protection, and if you are peri-menopausal and not yet out of the contraception business, a backup method, such as a birth control pill or an IUD, is a good choice.

3. Take one antibiotic pill after intercourse. Despite fears to the contrary, taking one antibiotic pill on a regular basis does not lead to an increase in yeast infections or antibiotic resistance.

4. Take a probiotic. A vaginal probiotic (taken orally) may help because increasing vaginal lactobacilli will theoretically prevent colonization of E.coli in the vagina. The science is not as solid, but preliminary data is encouraging!

If nothing you do seems to help, make an appointment

and see a urologist or urogynecologist to make sure that there isn't another reason for your recurrent infections.

But here is the real news you can use: If you are peri- or post-menopause, those recurrent bladder infections, along with that "gotta go" feeling even when you do not have an infection, are more likely than not a consequence of genitourinary syndrome of menopause. All the treatments for GSM described in chapters 6, 7, 8, and 9 will help you maintain a healthy vaginal microbiome, which translates to fewer bladder infections. Many of my patients have literally eliminated recurrent urinary infections by treating their vaginal dryness.

So if there is a persistent foul odor despite normal hygiene or if you are getting recurrent bladder infections or vulvar burning and irritation, skip the trip down the feminine hygiene aisle, and take a trip to your doctor instead. ▼

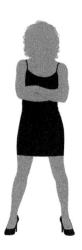

> NOW THAT COCONUT oil is off the table (and out of Francey's vagina), Francey notices that, more often than not, sex is less than pleasurable. She is a little mystified since she assumed things would improve now that she is having regular sex. (Use it or lose it!) She consults Dr. Google and is dismayed to learn that once vaginal dryness sets in, things tend to get worse with time, not better. She makes another appointment with her doctor, who is very sympathetic to her situation. Her doctor confirms that Francey has vaginal atrophy (yikes!) but also assures her that this is a normal part of aging. She suggests a bubble bath and a couple of glasses of wine before sexual activity. Francey, being no fool (and now a loyal patient of Dr. Google), decides she also needs a lubricant and heads off to the corner drugstore, where she grabs the first bottle she sees and, for good measure, a bag of chocolate-covered almonds big enough to hide the lube in her basket (in case she runs into anyone she knows).

4

THE LOWDOWN ON LUBES

MOST DRUGSTORES HAVE a dizzying selection of personal lubricants that promise everything from making things more slippery to increasing libido. There are shelves of vaginal lubricants that warm up, light up, and come with a theme song. It's daunting to say the least, which is why most women who find themselves experiencing sandpaper sex generally first head to the bathroom to see what they have on hand.

Slippery Stuff From Your Medicine Cabinet

Good old petroleum jelly might seem like a good idea, but it's not. Not only is it just about impossible to wash off, but the jelly also makes infection and irritation far more likely. In fact, one study showed that women who routinely put petroleum jelly inside their vagina were more than twice as likely to develop bacterial vaginosis. In addition, petroleum products cause deterioration of latex, as in condoms, which in turn increases the risk of acquiring sexually transmitted infections. In other words, petroleum jelly is fine for the lips on your face, not the lips of your vulva.

Baby oil is another popular choice. Good for baby's bottom, why not good for your bottom? Like petroleum jelly, baby oil can cause vaginal irritation and is associated with latex condom breakage. Oil-based products are also associated with a high rate of vaginal yeast infections.

Better for Making Lunch Than for Making Love

After women exhaust what's in their medicine cabinet, they often head on down to the kitchen. Why not just slather on a little olive oil, butter, vegetable shortening, coconut oil, almond oil, or apricot oil? Here's why. Like petroleum jelly, cooking oils dissolve latex and shouldn't be used with condoms. They don't work particularly well because their consistency is very thin. I also don't really see the allure of your vagina smelling like olive oil. And, again, regular use of oil in the vagina may increase the risk of a yeast infection. In other words, olive oil is great to use when making lunch, not when making love.

Bottom line: Petroleum jelly, baby oil, and cooking oils are fine to use in a pinch but should not be your regular go-to choices.

The Savvy Woman's Guide to Buying a Lubricant

When it comes to going to the drugstore, most women resort to one of two strategies. Either they grab the first product they see then stock up on shampoo and deodorant to hide the fact that vaginal lubricant is the only thing on their list in case they run into someone they know, or they grab a product they have seen advertised. Women willing to linger often pick the brand that promises the most. Inevitably, the results are disappointing.

The truth of the matter: Not all lubricants are created equal. So here is what will do what it is supposed to do.

A lubricant is defined as a substance that provides a slippery barrier between a penis or toy and vaginal tissue. Lubricants do not change or heal tissue. A lubricant decreases friction. Period.

There are three basic categories of commercially available lubes: water-based, silicone-based, and oil-based. Hybrid lubes combine water and silicone.

Water-Based Lubes

Water is interesting in that it can be really slippery (think slipping on a thin pool of it as you step out of the shower), but if there is a lot of friction, water can make things tacky or sticky. In addition to the fact that water-based lubes tend to be gloppy and sticky and simply don't last very long, most popular water-based lubes can, with continued use, damage and dehydrate vaginal tissue. Here's why:

Most water-based lubes contain glycerin and other additives to keep things on the slippery side. Another ingredient often found in many, but not all, water-based lubes is a preservative known as propylene glycol. Glycerin, propylene glycol, and other additives often found in water-based lubricants increase a product's osmolality.

A quick trip back to seventh grade science is needed to understand why this is a problem (I'll keep this short).

Osmolality is the measure of dissolved particles per unit of water in a solution. Water has an osmolality of zero. The vagina normally has a low osmolality, around 300 mOmol/kg, so you want whatever you're using to be as close as possible to that number.

If you put a lubricant with a high osmolality in the vagina, the vaginal cells will push water outside of the cells in an attempt to maintain a low vaginal osmolality. So lubricants with high osmolality not only dry out tissue (the opposite of what you are trying to accomplish!) but also increase the chance of irritation and infection because the tissue becomes damaged. Hence, the irritation, burning, and itching that many women experience with regular use

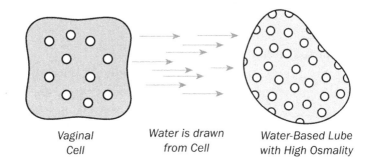

Vaginal
Cell

Water is drawn
from Cell

Water-Based Lube
with High Osmality

of many popular water-based lubricants.

The World Health Organization (WHO) recommends that vaginal lubricants should have an osmolality less than 1,200. If you are impressed that the WHO cares about dry vaginas, don't be. They don't care. What they do care about is transmission of sexually transmitted infections, and they have determined that lubricants with high osmolality increase the likelihood of acquiring HIV because of tissue damage and breakdown, which leaves a convenient entry portal for bacteria and viruses.

It's truly shocking how many of the most popular lubricants have a sky-high osmolality. There are newer lubricants that have a low osmolality, but you need to look for them. As a sweeping generalization, if a lubricant does not list its osmolality, it probably is off-the-charts high.

Many women avoid lubricants with glycerin, because they think they will cause yeast infections, and parabens, because they are concerned they will cause cancer (not true). The reason to avoid water-based lubes with those additives is that along with the additives comes a high osmolality.

OSMOLALITY OF COMMON WATER-BASED LUBRICANTS

(Ideally osmolality should be about 300 mOsm/kg and should never be greater than 1,200 mOsm/kg.)

K-Y Warming Jelly™ . . . . 10,300 mOsm/kg

Astroglide Liquid™ . . . . 8,000 mOsm/kg

Astroglide Silken Secret™ . . . . 6,000 mOsm/kg

K-Y Tingling Jelly™ . . . . 5,000 mOsm/kg

Liquid Silk™ . . . . 3,000 mOsm/kg

K-Y Jelly™ . . . . 2,000 mOsm/kg

Pjur Nude™ . . . . 2,000 mOsm/kg

Sylk Natural™ . . . . 847 mOsm/kg

Pulse H2Oh!™ . . . . 300 mOsm/kg

Good Clean Love™ . . . . 240 mOsm/kg

System Jo™ . . . . 61 mOsm/kg

Slippery Stuff™ . . . . 32 mOsm/kg

What About pH?

If the goal of a vaginal lubricant is to be as close as possible to vaginal secretions in terms of osmolality, then it stands to reason that a lubricant should also have a pH in the neighborhood of ~ 3.5-5.0 to maintain a healthy microbiome.

Silicone lubricants do not have a pH value, since they have no water. Water based lubricants vary in pH, and like osmolality, rarely advertise the pH level unless it is low. Having said that, pH is less than an issue when choosing a lubricant since unlike osmolality, which is often in the sky high tissue damaging range, the pH of most lubricants is between 3.0 and 6.0. Having said that, if you are someone that gets frequent bacterial vaginosis, you should make sure your lubricant is not the culprit that is killing off the healthy lactobacilli.

Silicone Lubricants

The tradeoff of using low osmolality water-based lubes is that, although they are non-irritating to vaginal tissue, they may not be slippery enough, or last long enough. (All of those osmolality increasing additives are what make them slippery.) Silicone lubricants, on the other hand, are very slippery, long- lasting, and non-irritating. In addition to being far more slippery than a water-based lubricant, silicone lubricants do not have osmolality or pH issues because they do not require preservatives or other irritating ingredients.

Silicone lubricants do not destroy latex and are condom-compatible. Because they don't break down in water, they are by far the best choice if you like having sex in the sauna, tub, or shower. A word of caution: If you are a fan of sex in the shower, beware that silicone lube on your shower floor translates to a high risk of slipping and falling. Try explaining that one to the paramedics!

The downside to silicone lubricants is that they are generally more expensive. But remember: A little bit goes a long way, and your vagina is worth it! Another minor negative is that for those without a flesh-and-blood man on hand, silicone lubes have the potential to react with silicone vaginal toys. Prolonged contact can cause the toy to become gummy or sticky, and in some cases, they can cause the silicone covering to swell and become misshapen. An easy workaround is to put a condom over your toy to protect it or simply wash the toy as soon as you are finished using it.

Also, silicone lubes can stain the sheets. If there is a stain, a concentrated stain remover will usually take care of it. Not to mention, it's not as if you'll be lying in a pool of the stuff. A lubricant generally stays where you put it: on his penis and in your vagina. Water-based-lube manufacturers make a big deal out of the fact that their products don't stain, but I have yet to have a patient tell me that silicone lubes are unacceptable because they ruin the sheets. Not to mention, it is far better to ruin the sheets than to ruin your sex life.

So where do you get silicone lubricants? Your local drugstore does carry them, but because of the higher price point, they may not have a huge selection. The internet is also a great way to find a selection of silicone lubes. Just be sure to specify silicone vaginal lubricant in your search or you are likely to come up with products meant for your carburetor.

And for the really thrifty shopper, there are a number of other uses for your silicone lube that have nothing to do with your genitals. Smear it all over your finger to get off that too-tight ring. Quiet a squeaky door. Polish your shoes. It's great for massages. And, yes, you can even use a dab of silicone lubricant on your hair to make it smooth and shiny. It turns out, the silicone product you put in your hair is essentially the same stuff that is manufactured to use as a vaginal lubricant. Just don't use an item intended for your hair in your vagina because the hair products have perfumes, which can be irritating.

Oil-Based Lubricants

There are a handful of commercial lubricants that are oil-based rather than silicon- or water-based. Oil-based lubricants are not condom-compatible. They are also ... oily. Some women like them because they are thinner and feel more like the real deal. Although there are no studies that actually compare the various types of lubes, I have yet to have a patient tell me that an oil-based lube lasted as long or was as slippery as a silicone product.

Getting It Where It Needs to Go

Most products come with excruciatingly detailed instructions even when it is pretty obvious how they should be used. You really don't need to be told to rinse the shampoo out of your hair, but the back of the shampoo bottle always tells you specifically to do so.

Lubricant, on the other hand, comes instruction-free despite the fact that a lot of women are not really sure when or how to use it. When you are in "the moment" is probably not the best time to try to figure it out.

First, I suggest you remove the packaging and put the lube in a handy place well in advance of when you expect to use it. You don't want to go on the hunt. Once you are in the moment, if there is any chance—any chance!—that you will be dry and you think you are going to need some lubricant, do not try to have intercourse without applying it to "see how it goes." I can guarantee you, it is not going to go well.

And once you try to experience the agony of sandpaper sex, it's pretty much game over. Your vagina is not stupid, which means that the muscles surrounding the vagina will go into protective mode to prevent another painful attempt. When pelvic muscles spasm and tighten, the vaginal opening will be constricted, and the tissue will become even drier than usual. Once that happens, you can pretty much forget it. A bathtub full of lube is not going to help.

So slather the lubricant on you and your partner (or toy) before you start. The worst that will happen is that it will be too slippery. The easiest approach is to put a generous amount of lube on your (or his) fingers and apply it to the opening of your vagina. Coat his penis in it as well. (I guarantee he will like this part.) His penis will be the delivery system to the inside of your vagina.

Some women use a "lube shooter," or a small cylinder with a plunger that is inserted in the vagina in order to squirt lube inside. This is also a strategy to use if for some reason you don't want him to know that your slippery moisture is not all "you," and you want to apply it in the bathroom before things get going.

It's also nice to warm lubricant before use because it is less than pleasant to put cold stuff on genitals. There are a number of commercial lubricant warmers. Some let you use the lube of your choice; others require you to use the lube that goes with the device. If you are a planner, you can go low-tech and immerse your bottle of lubricant in a warm water bath in your sink before applying.

"Special" Lubes

Water and silicone based lubricants can often turn sandpaper sex into slippery sex. But for those who are also hoping their lube will take their sexual activity to a whole new level, enter specialty lubes.

Flavored Lubricants

Cookies and cream, sun-ripened strawberry, chocolate-raspberry, passion fruit, cinnamon, wild cherry, kiwi-strawberry, lemon-lime, hot strawberry, orange-mango, watermelon (no seeds!), bubble gum, and raspberry kiss. Ben & Jerry, eat your hearts out.

There are three reasons you might buy a flavored lubricant:

1. One is that you have an unpleasant vaginal odor you are trying to cover up. If that is the case, find out why there is an odor, and make it go away.

2. The second reason is if the man in your life doesn't like the way a normal vagina tastes or smells. Although that's his problem, his problem becomes your problem. And if that's the only way he will agree to oral sex, so be it.

3. The third reason is that he loves the way you taste and smell, but you both think it would be "fun" to try a flavor. Some people even like to lick chocolate off each other's genitals. This goes in that category. And far be it from me to get in the way of fun.

Water-based flavored lubes are edible. Silicone-based flavored lubes are not considered edible, but if you swallow a little, doing so won't cause any harm.

Flavored lubricants are generally water-based and have a sky-high osmolality. Over time, they will dry out and irritate vaginal tissue. It's probably best to save flavored lube for special occasions.

Warming Lubricants

The idea behind warming lubricants is that, in addition to reducing friction, they intensify and increase pleasurable sensations. These lubes are not warm in terms of temperature; they are chemically intended to heat things up. An ingredient such as capsaicin, a component of chili peppers, causes the warming sensation. (I couldn't make this stuff up.)

There are no scientific studies that have determined whether warming lubricants actually have a positive sexual effect. Anecdotally, and not surprisingly, many of my patients report a stinging or burning with these products. But if you put chili peppers in your vagina, maybe you should expect some burning to be involved.

Warming lubricants have really, really high osmolality and should not be used on a regular basis. If you have problems with vaginal dryness or irritation, steer clear.

Kosher Lubricants

Orthodox Jews follow very strict laws regarding food

and drink. Not only are specific foods forbidden, but the preparation of food is also strictly regulated. On the other hand, things that are applied externally such as cosmetics, skin lotion or even lip balm, do not need to be kosher. Strictly speaking, vaginal lubricant does not need to be kosher, unless there is any, any, chance that it is ingested. In other words, for the most orthodox of Jews, oral sex was basically off the table if a lubricant was on the table. With that in mind, one lube went to the trouble to pass the stringent requirements necessary to bear the "kosher" stamp that observant Jews require for any product that is ingested. Wet™ lubricants "kosherized" their production plant and passed rabbinical inspection to ensure that none of Wet's products contain ingredients derived from pigs or shellfish, and that any other animals used to create the lubes were treated humanely.

As Rabbi Shmuley Boteach, author of the bestselling book Kosher Sex, says, "It's nice to see that rabbis are not shying away from addressing sexual aids, which will facilitate great excitement in the bedroom," he said. "People misunderstand Orthodox Jews, in that they believe that they have sex through a sheet with a hole in the middle, that Orthodoxy is profoundly prudish. Orthodoxy is profoundly passionate. Orthodox couples have great sex lives."

But, Rabbi Boteach may have been overly optimistic about Orthodox Jews embracing better sex given that one week after Wet™ received it's Kosher certification it was taken away since evidently the certification board was not aware that this lubricant was to be used for sexual purposes, and specifically, for oral sex. Were they thinking this was lubricant for Jewish carburetors? In any case, even without the "official" certification, for those that care, no pigs were used in the making of Wet™.

CBD for Your Vag?

CBD is in your smoothies, your chocolate, and your muscle balm—why not your lube? CBD lubes claim to not only decrease pain and irritation, but also to increase libido and the ability to have an orgasm. I have even seen claims that CBD applied to the vagina will eliminate PTSD from prior sexual trauma.

Here's the problem. There is no research. None. Zip. Any "research" that is cited is generally marketing research, or anecdotal testimonials, not scientific research. A typical marketing campaign reads, "We gave CBD lube to fifty women, and ninety-eight percent of them said it was awesome!" It sounds convincing, but in my world, you need to give lube to hundreds of women and do what is known as a "blinded" comparison, meaning fifty percent get lube with CBD, fifty percent get lube without CBD, and then you see if the CBD group has a benefit over the non-CBD group.

So in the absence of data, I'm not recommending CBD lube, but I am not *not* recommending CBD lube.

Here's what is known:

- Most CBD lubes are oil-based and not condom-compatible. There are some that are water- or silicone-based.
- CBD does have anti-inflammatory properties and may help with vulvar inflammation.
- CBD dilates blood vessels and increases blood supply, which, in theory, may help with lubrication.

What If You Are Using a Prescription Product to Help With Lubrication?

Many women who use one of the products I discuss in subsequent chapters assume they will no longer need a lubricant. That is not necessarily the case. Even if you are using an estrogen product, DHEA, ospemifene, or have had vaginal laser treatments, most women still need the slippery stuff.

In general, most of my patients tell me that a good silicone lube makes all the difference in the world. So splurge. Trust me, if you spring for the good lubricant, your vagina, your partner, and even your hair will thank you.

Advantages of Lubricants
- Lubricants are readily available over the counter.
- They do not need to be used on a regular basis or in anticipation of intercourse, only "in the moment."
- Silicone-based and some (but not all) water-based lubricants are risk-free and do not damage vaginal tissue.

Disadvantages of Lubricants
- They are not covered by insurance.
- Most popular water-based lubricants have a high osmolality and over time can be irritating, damage vaginal tissue, and cause dehydration, not lubrication.
- They work only in mild cases of genitourinary syndrome of menopause.
- Sometimes multiple applications are required during sexual activity.
- They can be messy and inconvenient.
- They do not treat any of the other symptoms of GSM other than pain with intercourse. ▼

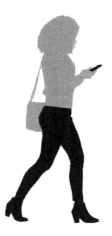

> THINGS ARE GOING fine until Francey's best friend informs her that she came across Adam's profile on Match.com. Being proactive, Francey decides to break up with him before he breaks up with her. Now more optimistic about new sexual experiences, she jumps online and quickly meets Kyle, who seems great, except for a snarky comment that only "old people need lubricant."

That should have been the tip-off that Kyle was a world-class jerk, but he did have other qualities, like giving world-class foot massages, so Francey opts to stick it out. After consulting with Dr. Google about an alternative to lubricant, she decides to try a long-acting vaginal moisturizer that can be applied in advance.

The moisturizer definitely helps, but over time she realizes that she also needs to use some lube. While on Amazon deciding between a silicone- and a water-based option, she also impulsively buys a shiatsu foot massager—and that is the end of Kyle.

5

MOISTURIZERS ARE NOT JUST FOR YOUR FACE

THE BATTLE TO keep skin from succumbing to the ravages of time is a never-ending, exhausting process—a battle fought through the regular slathering of moisturizer on your face, neck, legs, and vagina. Vagina? Although the "skin" that lines the vagina is not the same as the skin on the rest of your body, as estrogen declines, the vaginal cells shrink and become dehydrated, contributing to post-menopause, paper-thin, dry tissue. However, simply putting water in the vagina won't do the trick any more than washing your face will prevent wrinkles. The challenge of a *true* vaginal moisturizer is to get the cells that line the vaginal walls to suck the water in.

A Moisturizer Is NOT a Lubricant

Let's start with the fact that vaginal moisturizers and lubricants are not the same thing. Lubricants do not alter vaginal tissues; they just provide a slippery barrier to reduce friction at the time of intercourse. A moisturizer, on the other hand, is intended to change the water content of the cells (hence "moisturizer"), resulting in tissues that are more elastic, are thicker, and have the enhanced ability to produce fluid. A true long-acting moisturizer is used in anticipation of intercourse, not at the time of intercourse.

Here's where it gets confusing. Just because a product is labeled as a moisturizer, don't assume that it is going to hydrate vaginal tissues. The majority of products that are labeled as "personal" or "feminine" moisturizers are not even intended to be put inside the vagina. These products have no long-acting effect on vaginal walls or vaginal lubrication. They are actually intended to lubricate or soften vulvar tissue outside the vagina, but you would never know that from the way the products are labeled.

Just as a face cream can promise to make you look ten years younger with regular use, a "feminine" moisturizer can claim to make intercourse more comfortable. Unlike with prescription medications, the companies that market these products are under no obligation to the Food and Drug Administration to conduct scientific studies to prove that a product does what it claims to do. (See chapter 11 for more information on the role of the FDA when it comes to marketing!)

In addition, if a lubricant is labeled "for vaginal use," the FDA requires specific safety trials, including testing the product in animal vaginas to ensure that there are no harmful effects. This is a boon for the rats that suffer from vaginal dryness, but it adds an enormous expense to product development. It's cheaper and easier for manufacturers to just avoid the word "vagina" altogether on their labeling.

In addition, many lubricants that are intended to go inside the vagina are labeled as "moisturizers" because manufacturers think that makes the products sound more appealing. Purchasing a "feminine moisturizer" is far more comfortable for women who are also buying a hand moisturizer and a face moisturizer than it would be

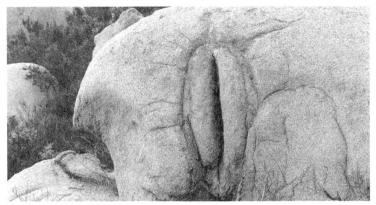

The surface of your vulva should never resemble the dry and cracked surface of this actual rock formation that I came upon while hiking Mount Kuchamaa at Rancho La Puerta.

for them to go shopping for a "lube" that is clearly intended for sexual purposes. The manufacturers are operating under the assumption that *"nice, church-going, married women buy moisturizers. Hussies buy lubes."* It's misleading and confusing—and it works.

The only true *vaginal* moisturizers are products that are meant to be inserted inside the vagina to increase the water content of cells so that the vaginal walls produce more natural lubrication. Any product labeled "for external use only" is NOT a vaginal moisturizer.

Two kinds of over-the-counter options have been shown in scientific clinical studies to actually change vaginal tissue, increase intracellular water, and decrease painful intercourse: Replens Long Lasting Vaginal Moisturizer™ and products that contain hyaluronic acid, such as Hyalo Gyn Vaginal Hydrating Gel™ and Revaree Hyaluronic Acid Ovules™.

How Long-Acting Moisturizers Work

Replens Long Acting Vaginal Moisturizer™ contains

47

polycarbophil, a bio-adhesive gel that adheres to the vaginal wall and promotes intracellular water absorption. Polycarbophil is also a weak acid that buffers vaginal tissues to lower the vaginal pH to between 3 and 4.5, allowing repopulation of lactobacilli (healthy vaginal bacteria). Most important, it has been shown in scientific clinical trials to increase vaginal elasticity and lubrication.

Hyaluronic acid vaginal gels and suppositories are the other category of over-the-counter long-acting moisturizers that are used to alleviate vaginal dryness. Hyaluronic acid is naturally produced by the body in the skin, connective tissue, and eyes and works by binding to water to retain moisture. Although commonly used to prevent wrinkles in skin, it has also been found useful in increasing wrinkles in your vaginal wall. (Remember, vaginal wrinkles are a good thing!) In a small clinical trial, hyaluronic acid worked as well as estriol (a weak form of estrogen), but not as well as topical estradiol, to relieve vaginal itching, burning, and painful intercourse.

I am often asked which type of product works better. There have been no scientific studies that compare the two options. I can tell you anecdotally that both work well, and it is a matter of personal preference.

How to Use a Long-Acting Moisturizer

Consistency is critical. If you use one only once in a while or in anticipation of weekend sexual activity, don't bother. Like all products to restore vaginal tissue, these products are only effective if used regularly.

And though the product instructions recommend twice-weekly use, many women need to use one more frequently: up to four times per week. This is particularly the case if someone is going through chemotherapy. Be sure and take some of the gel and apply it to the vestibule, the opening of the vagina. And, yes, you will most likely still need to use a lubricant at the time of intercourse.

Advantages of Long-Acting Vaginal Moisturizers
- They are readily available over the counter, so no visit to the doctor and no prescription required.
- They're hormone-free.
- The gel can be applied to the vestibule as well.

Disadvantages of Long Acting Moisturizers
- Moisturizers are not covered by insurance and over time can be expensive.
- Moisturizers work best in cases of mild atrophy.
- They require consistent twice-weekly application, but sometimes greater frequency is necessary.
- They can be messy, and there is an occasional discharge.
- Many women find that a long-acting moisturizer is all that they need to alleviate vaginal dryness. Having said that, if you do not get relief, you may have to bite the bullet and go to your doctor to get a prescription product. ▼

❯ *WHAT A RELIEF to be hanging out with*
female friends! Francey and her besties
haven't even finished their second glass of
wine when the vagina talk starts. When
Francey brings up her quest for the return of
her 30-year-old vagina, Shari is floored that Francey's doctor
hasn't even mentioned the option of vaginal estrogen. She's
personally a big fan of the estrogen ring that requires her to
think about the fact that her vagina has entered menopause
only every three months.

Annoyed that her own doctor has not brought it up,
Francey makes an appointment with Shari's doctor. Though
there is no penis in her life at the moment, she wants to
be ready for when she does meet someone new, and she's
intrigued by not having to think about her vagina every day.

6

ESTROGEN RINGS, CREAMS
AND OTHER THINGS

IT WOULD BE nice if lubricants always solved the problem. But sometimes the ravages of menopause make the vaginal walls so thin and dry that the only way to reverse the vaginal clock and make intercourse comfortable is to bite the bullet, go to a doctor, and get a prescription for a medication that will restore your vaginal walls to their glory days. At the top of the list of prescription products is estrogen. Makes sense: It was your lack of estrogen that caused the problem in the first place.

Local vaginal estrogens are products that are placed in the vagina to specifically alleviate the symptoms of genitourinary syndrome of menopause. What that means is, not only will a local vaginal estrogen restore normal elasticity and lubrication, but there is also a good chance that it will alleviate irritation, urinary urgency, and recurrent urinary tract infections. In other words, penetrative sexual activity doesn't need to be on the menu for you to benefit.

Estrogen works, and estrogen is safe. But you wouldn't know it from reading the FDA-required package insert that practically has a skull and crossbones on it, causing you to consider if it is really worth getting breast cancer, dementia, heart disease, or a stroke just to have a decent orgasm. Except nothing written on that warning is true, and there is no need to update your will before you start to treat your vaginal dryness. Here's the deal:

FDA class labeling requires all products containing the same ingredient to have the same warning, even if the issue has never been demonstrated in that product. For example, taking oral systemic estrogens can increase the risk of developing a blood clot. That risk has never been demonstrated in the use of a local vaginal estrogen product; nevertheless, the FDA requires that warning to be on every product that contains estrogen. In fact, every single one of the warnings on local vaginal estrogen labels is based on the risks associated with systemic oral estrogen. Not one single complication listed on the package insert has ever been shown to result from using vaginal estrogen. On the contrary, there are multiple scientific studies that confirm that use of local vaginal estrogen does not increase the risk of blood clots, cancer, dementia, or cancer.

Some vaginal estrogen is absorbed into the bloodstream, but the amount is minimal, and its effects are local rather than systemic. Just to keep it in perspective, the amount of systemic absorption of estrogen in a full year of using a local vaginal estrogen is roughly the same as if you took one birth control tablet a year. Blood levels of women who use vaginal estrogen are no different than those of post-menopause women who do not use vaginal estrogen.

For that reason, vaginal estrogen has no impact on your hot flashes, bones, or brain. And for the same reason, local vaginal estrogen is safe to use even if you have breast cancer or a history of blood clots.

Phew. Now let's get down to the details.

THE PRODUCTS

When it comes to local vaginal estrogen products, you

have a lot of choices. All are safe, all are effective, and all require a prescription. Dosing is usually based on increased frequency for initial therapy (to repair the tissue), followed by less intense maintenance therapy. Consistency is critical to success, and if you stop using a product, all the benefits will be lost. The choice of estrogen is a combination of personal preference, what works best for you, and, sadly, cost and insurance coverage.

I also want to emphasize that none of the manufacturers of these products have paid to be included in this guide, and I am including all the prescription products currently available.

VAGINAL ESTROGEN CREAMS
Product names:
>Estrace™ *(estradiol .01%)*,
>Premarin™ *(conjugated estrogens)*

How they're used: The creams come in a toothpaste-like tube. You squeeze one into a reusable applicator, insert the applicator into the vagina, and use a plunger to release the cream. The typical recommended dosage is one half to one full applicator. There are a number of protocols, but in general, the cream is used daily for 14 days and then maintained with twice-weekly use.

For women who prefer not to use an applicator, another option is to put a strip of cream on your finger and insert your finger into your vagina—environmentally friendly, and no applicator to wash and reuse! The cream can also be directly applied on the outside of the vagina to the tissue of the vulva, vestibule, and clitoris. If you are experiencing urinary symptoms such as urgency, or frequency, a dab of estrogen cream applied directly to the urethra often helps alleviate those symptoms.

Advantages

- Creams are generally the least expensive form of vaginal estrogen because they have been around a long time.
- You can taper the amount of cream you insert to determine the lowest amount you need to get results. The advantage of using the lowest amount of cream has nothing to do with safety. The advantage is that it is less expensive and not as messy.
- Cream can also be applied directly to the opening or outside of the vagina to help reverse thinness and dryness of external tissues such as the vulva, vestibule, and clitoris.
- A tiny amount of estrogen cream applied to the urethra often eliminates urinary symptoms such as urgency or recurrent urinary tract infections.
- Bonus! Creams can be applied directly to the clitoris to increase blood flow for help having orgasms.

Disadvantages

- Creams tend to be messy. They tend to "drip" out of the vagina.
- Loading the applicator is an extra step.
- The reusable applicator, while environmentally friendly, has to be washed after every use. Although putting it in the dishwasher is efficient, other members of the household may object.
- For some, the twice-weekly schedule is an opportunity to forget to use the product, twice a week.

Premarin™ issues:

○ Horse lover alert! Premarin™ is produced from the urine of pregnant horses (PREgnant MARe urINe—get it?). Many women object to the way the horses aretreated in collecting said urine and boycott this product.

- All of the other estrogen products are plant-derived, "bio-identical" estrogen, (meaning it is structurally identical to the estrogen naturally produced by ovaries) so women looking for something "natural" often avoid Premarin™ because it is not plant-derived. I have three things to say about this: One, what could be more natural than horse piss? Two, humans are closer to horses than plants. Three, natural isn't always safe. Arsenic comes to mind.

VAGINAL ESTROGEN RING
Product name:

Estring™ *(estradiol vaginal ring-2 mg)*
(Note: Femring™ is also an estrogen ring, but it delivers higher, systemic dosages of estrogen intended for the treatment of hot flashes.)

How it's used: It is a flexible, silastic, disposable ring that you insert into the vagina and replace every three months. The ring slowly releases tiny amounts of estradiol and is one size fits all. You simply fold the flexible 2-inch ring and give it a little push so it slips into the back of the vagina. Once it is in, you will not feel it or be aware of it in any way. It does not need to be removed during intercourse (although you can if you want to), and it is only the rare guy who can feel it. When it's time for removal, you use your fingers to pull it out.

Advantages
- Convenience, convenience, convenience. You need to think about this product only four times a year.

- There is no dripping cream.
- There is no applicator to load, wash, or hide.

Disadvantages
- An internal ring offers some vulvar benefits but not as many as estrogen creams.
- You cannot taper the amount of estrogen being delivered the way you can with estrogen creams.
- Some women just don't like having something inside their vagina all the time.
- Some women have difficulty putting it in place.
- Some women find it difficult to remove. I do have a handful of patients who come in and have me do it for them. Alternatively, you can tie a length of dental floss ribbon (unminted!) to the ring, tuck the floss into your vagina once you place the ring, and, when it is time for removal, fish out the floss and use it to pull the ring down so it is easily reachable.

VAGINAL ESTROGEN TABLETS
Product names:
Vagifem™, Uvafem™, and other generics
(*estradiol 10 mcg*)

How they're used: The tiny tablets (about the size of a baby aspirin) come preloaded on a slender disposable applicator. You insert the applicator a few inches into the vagina, push the plunger to release a tablet, and then throw 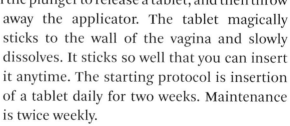 away the applicator. The tablet magically sticks to the wall of the vagina and slowly dissolves. It sticks so well that you can insert it anytime. The starting protocol is insertion of a tablet daily for two weeks. Maintenance is twice weekly.

Advantages
- The applicator is pre-loaded, so there is no "prep."
- The tablets release a consistent dose of estrogen.
- Not messy.
- Easy to use.
- There's no applicator to load, wash, or hide.
- You can use the tablets AM or PM.
- The tablets deliver a lower dose of estrogen than the creams or ring. That doesn't make them any safer (they are all equally safe). But for women who desire the lowest dose of estrogen, this and the estradiol insert (see below) are the ones.

Disadvantages
- Vaginal tablets primarily deliver internal benefits and in many of my patients inadequately treat the vestibule and vaginal opening.
- This product only comes in one dose which is too low for many women.
- For some, the twice-weekly schedule is an opportunity to forget to use the product, twice a week.
- Environmentally conscious women don't like that the disposable applicator is not biodegradable. Twice-weekly use starting at age 50 and continuing to age 90 is approximately 3,500 applicators—basically a small mountain.

VAGINAL ESTROGEN INSERTS
Product name:
  Imvexxy™ (*estradiol 4 mcg, 10 mcg*)

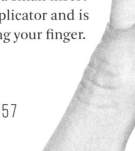

How it's used: Imvexxy™ is a small insert that does not require an applicator and is pushed into the vagina using your finger.

The starting dose is every night for two weeks. Maintenance is twice weekly.

Advantages
- Inserts deliver a consistent dose of estrogen.
- The amount of systemic absorption of estradiol is even lower than the already extremely low absorption with vaginal tablet use.
- There are two doses available.
- Not messy.
- Easy to use.
- There's no applicator to load, wash, or hide.
- It can be used AM or PM.

Disadvantages
- Vaginal inserts primarily deliver internal benefits and in some of my patients are inadequate when it comes to treating the vestibule and vaginal opening.
- For some, the twice-weekly schedule is an opportunity to forget to use the product, twice a week.

AFTER HEARING ALL of her options, Francey decides to go the ring route. But when she goes to pick it up at the pharmacy, she learns that it isn't covered by her insurance. She doesn't want to take a second job to pay for her sex life, so she opts for her second choice, the generic version of the estradiol vaginal tablet.

Leaving the pharmacy carrying her new prescription, she decides to celebrate the imminent rebirth of her vagina with a manicure. Feeling a bit like a vagina evangelist, she can't wait to tell her longtime manicurist, Val, who is her age, all about the wonders of vaginal estrogen. But Val's reaction quickly bursts that bubble; she proclaims that if Francey uses vaginal estrogen, she will definitely get breast cancer and die. "That's exactly what happened to my brother's wife's best friend just weeks after she started using vaginal estrogen," she says as she trims Francey's cuticles.

Francey again consults Dr. Google, who honestly doesn't make her feel any better. As luck would have it, she matches with Steve, who happens to be, of all things, a breast surgeon. Not one to pass up the opportunity for a free consultation, she agrees to meet him for a drink. Over a glass of chardonnay, while trying not to stare at the tiny piece of lettuce stuck between his front teeth, she asks his opinion on the use of vaginal estrogen. He, assuming that Francey's inquiry is a prelude to having sex with him, enthusiastically gives her a far-too-detailed lecture on the safety of using it.

At the end of the evening, she concludes two things: One, she does not want to go on a second date with Steve, and, two, she needs a new manicurist who is not so opinionated.

The vaginal pill is certainly easy to use, but Francey is still noticing that the opening of her vagina is dry, even when she is having sex with her toy. Everything is fine once it's inside, but getting it in feels like someone has sprinkled ground glass at the opening of her vagina. Wishing her doctor had a frequent-flyer plan, she makes yet another appointment to find out why the vaginal pill isn't working. After an exam, the doctor proclaims that the pill is working just fine inside her vagina, but her vestibule is still dry. The solution, she says, is to apply an estrogen cream a couple of times per week to the area surrounding the opening of her vagina in addition to inserting the vaginal pill.

The Best
of Both Worlds
—*or*—
It doesn't matter how nice the room is if you can't get through the door

FOR MANY WOMEN, an estrogen tablet, ring, or insert placed in the vagina does a great job restoring vaginal lubrication and elasticity. But it doesn't do much of anything for the opening of the vagina. In fact, the majority of treatment "failures" I see in women who are using an estrogen product is that the product is only adequately treating the inside. Using a cream solves the dryness problem, but there is the mess, the applicator, etc. The solution is to do a combo approach: Use a ring, tablet, or insert to get rid of the internal sandpaper feeling, and apply a small dab of estrogen cream on the vestibule and vulva once or twice a week.

FAQ About Local Vaginal Estrogen

I went through menopause 20 years ago. Is it too late to start?

The perfect time to start is … anytime. Systemic estrogen to treat hot flashes should ideally be started within the first few years of menopause. Vaginal estrogen is different. It is safe and effective to start even decades after your last period. There is research that indicates that the earlier you begin, the more effective it will be. But I have had patients who were well into their 80s when they started treatment, and they did just fine.

I use an estrogen patch. Will that get rid of vaginal dryness?

Maybe. Systemic estrogens such as pills, sprays, patches, and skin gels are intended to work throughout the body to alleviate symptoms such as hot flashes. One vaginal product, Femring™, provides systemic levels of estrogen. In about 75% of cases, systemic estrogen relieves vaginal dryness and additional local vaginal estrogen is not needed. And, yes, you can use a local vaginal estrogen product along with your estrogen patch.

How long can I (or should I) use vaginal estrogen?

Hot flashes are fleeting, but dryness is forever. If you stop, it's pretty much a guarantee that the dryness will return. So, you should use vaginal estrogen as long as you're interested in having intercourse and maintaining vaginal and urinary health—in other words, until death. The real challenge is finding a partner who is still "good to go."

And not to worry: Estrogen does not accumulate over time. The blood level of estrogen in a woman who has been using local estrogen for two years is the same as it is in a woman who has been using it for ten years. The North American Menopause Society (NAMS) has issued a position statement that says, "Vaginal estrogen therapy should be continued as long as distressful symptoms remain."

If my male partner gets estrogen on his penis,
will he grow breasts?

No. Next question.

I am going on vacation with my new boyfriend.
How quickly does it work?

Pretty quick, but probably not quick enough for you. Within two to four weeks of initiating local estrogen therapy, most women are able to have comfortable intercourse. In fact, a look at vaginal tissue under a microscope shows that normal thickness is often restored to the vaginal walls in that amount of time, and the tissue is indistinguishable from pre-menopausal vaginal tissue. Some women need a longer "repair" time, and the effects are cumulative.

Will I still need to use a lubricant?
Yes. Next question.

Should I continue to use vaginal estrogen
if I am between partners?
If you stop your estrogen treatment, it doesn't take long for atrophy to set in again. In other words, skipping your estrogen for months and then deciding to use it the night before you leave on a cruise is not a good plan. Vaginal estrogen products are not lubricants—they restore lubrication. There is no reason to stop (other than convenience and cost), and if you take a hiatus, it may take a month to get things back in shape. In addition to keeping up with your vaginal estrogen, it's also a good idea if you are between partners to stimulate vaginal tissue using a dildo or vibrator. There is truth to use it or lose it.

Should I use vaginal estrogen if I am not
interested in having sex?
Often women who are between partners, or not interested in sexual activity for whatever reason, ask if they should continue to use vaginal estrogen. That depends. Many women use vaginal estrogen for nonsexual benefits, such as preventing recurrent urinary tract infections and reducing or eliminating urinary urgency. Other post-menopause women experience chronic itching and irritation from dryness and are just far more comfortable using a

local vaginal estrogen in the vagina or on the vulva. But if you have no urinary symptoms and no genital discomfort, there is no reason to use vaginal estrogen.

What if I have breast cancer?

Stay tuned for Dr. Streicher's Inside Information on Sex and Cancer for all the details, but here's the headline: There is no evidence that using local vaginal estrogen directly causes an increased risk of breast cancer recurrence. On the contrary, there is a lot of reassuring data that proves the exact opposite. One study of 1,472 breast cancer patients who routinely used vaginal estrogen determined that women with breast cancer who used estrogen had a lower recurrence rate than women who did not use vaginal estrogen. In 2016, the American College of Obstetricians and Gynecologists (ACOG) released a position statement very clearly stating that the use of estrogen in women with breast cancer is safe and appropriate. Having said that, subsequent chapters talk about non-estrogen options.

What about testosterone cream?

Vaginal and vulvar tissues are rich in testosterone receptors that play a role in normal lubrication. Vaginal testosterone is not FDA approved and therefore not available commercially. In cases of severe vulvar and vaginal atrophy, I and many other experts prescribe testosterone cream alone or in combination with estrogen which can be compounded and prescribed for this purpose. ▼

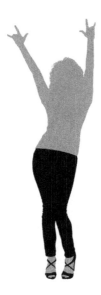

❯ *AFTER QUITE THE dry spell (as in dating, not vaginas), Francey meets Randy, an incredibly normal guy who is fun, smart, and sexy and does not need a map to her clitoris. Things are going great, but after she tells Randy her vagina regimen (estrogen tablet twice weekly, estrogen cream twice weekly, and plenty of lube during sex), he mentions that the last woman in his life used a DHEA suppository that not only provided great lubrication but also seemed to boost her libido. Being a team player, Francey agrees to give it a try.*

7

DHEA-HEY HEY!

MOST SAVVY WOMEN are well aware that estrogen is a key ingredient to ensure vaginal elasticity and lubrication. But less appreciated is that testosterone receptors are also present in vaginal and vulvar tissues and also contribute to lubrication and elasticity. Didehydroepiandrosterone, or DHEA, is the building block that our bodies require to manufacture both estrogen and testosterone. Women naturally have their own supply of DHEA, thoughtfully provided by the adrenal glands. But here's the bad news (you knew this was coming): Adrenal DHEA decreases by roughly sixty percent at menopause and continues to decline over time.

Enter a non-estrogen prescription alternative to treat vaginal dryness: DHEA vaginal suppositories, also known as prasterone. Prasterone /DHEA has been prescribed for years by menopause experts but needed to be compounded by a specialty pharmacy because there was no commercial product available. In 2016, the FDA approved prasterone (trade name Intrarosa™) specifically for the treatment of women experiencing moderate to severe pain during sex.

This once-daily vaginal insert has been shown to have all the effects of a local vaginal estrogen, including increasing lubrication and elasticity and alleviating pain during intercourse. Like the local vaginal estrogen products, there is also a good chance that DHEA will alleviate irritation, urinary urgency, and recurrent urinary tract infections.

And bonus! DHEA may also enhance libido. Obviously, any treatment to alleviate painful sex will often boost an absent libido since most people don't want to do something painful. But interestingly, some studies show that women who use vaginal DHEA have an increase in sex drive and orgasm beyond what is expected from eliminating painful intercourse. This makes sense given that DHEA is a building block for both estrogen and testosterone. Since testosterone is not only important for vaginal and vulvar health but is also the 'I am thinking about sex and want to have sex" hormone, it follows that a bump might increase sex drive.

How Prasterone/DHEA Works

DHEA works inside vaginal cells and is converted to both estrogen and testosterone, which in turn increase vaginal lubrication and elasticity and decreases painful sex. Local DHEA supplementation is safe and does not increase systemic levels of estrogen or stimulate hormone receptors in breast or uterine tissue.

How You Use Prasterone/DHEA

Vaginal DHEA/prasterone is a bullet-shaped suppository that comes packaged in a blister pack. The suppository is placed in the lower third of the vagina using a reusable applicator, but most of my patients skip the applicator and just push it in with a finger. Once the suppository is placed in the vagina, your body temperature immediately causes it to melt. You might want to use this product at bedtime because there is a tendency for it to drip out if you are up and about. And speaking of melting, don't store it by a sunny window; it needs to be kept at room temperature. The company also states that it can be kept in the refrigerator, a real selling point because we all know how women love to put something really cold in their vagina. Not to mention, do you really want to keep your vaginal suppositories next to your eggs?

The only complaint I have heard is that some women say it makes them too juicy! And if that is the case, try every other day application.

Advantages

- It works as well, if not better, than vaginal estrogen because it also stimulates testosterone production.
- It is an excellent estrogen alternative.
Unlike with a vaginal estrogen tablet, because some of the medication leaks out, both the vagina and the vestibule are treated.
- It possibly increases libido and orgasm beyond what is expected from eliminating painful intercourse.

Disadvantages

- This product, like the local vaginal estrogens, requires requires vaginal insertion, which is a negative for many women.
- The daily dosing is inconvenient.
- Some women complain that it is messy because some of the medication drips out of the vagina when it melts.
- It must be stored between 41°F and 86°F.
- As with many new products, the cost is prohibitive if it's not covered by insurance. Prior to FDA approval

of this product, it could be compounded in specialty pharmacies. I still utilize this option for women who do not have insurance coverage.

- Although it is not estrogen, it is a precursor to estrogen, and some breast surgeons recommend avoidance, particularly in women taking aromatase inhibitors or tamoxifen.

FAQ About Prasterone/DHEA

Does prasterone/DHEA work better than local vaginal estrogen?

There are no head-to-head studies that definitively answer this question but given that it stimulates the local production of both estrogen and testosterone, it stands to reason that it might. Anecdotally, I have many patients who have better results with prasterone/DHEA than with local estrogen.

Is it safe for women with breast cancer?

For women concerned about minute amounts of estrogen entering their system, although the amount of estrogen produced by DHEA is ridiculously low, it is not zero. I maintain that vaginal estrogen is safe to use in women with breast cancer (see chapter 5!). Most breast surgeons and oncologists I work with are very comfortable with patients using vaginal DHEA. Having said that, if you are not comfortable with even a minute amount of estrogen, you may choose to go in a different direction.

There is also a theoretical concern that DHEA will decrease the effectiveness of hormonal chemotherapy medicines such as an aromatase inhibitor or tamoxifen. That has not been shown to be the case with DHEA used locally, but it is a reason why some breast experts discourage its use.

Do dietary supplements containing DHEA
help alleviate vaginal dryness?

DHEA supplements are really popular, which is hardly surprising when you read their list of benefits, including building up the adrenal glands, strengthening the immune system, anti-aging, increasing energy, balancing hormones, improving mood and memory, building bone and muscle strength, burning fat, and, yes, reversing vaginal dryness and pain. Impressive, and it makes me want to start taking some immediately! But this is yet another example of marketing trumping science. There are zero scientific studies that show that an oral DHEA has any benefits, despite the claims these companies make. There are also safety concerns. So the answer is, no, DHEA dietary supplements do not alleviate vaginal dryness. ▼

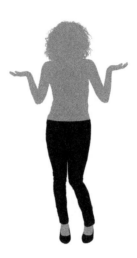

❯ *THINGS ARE STILL going great with Harry and they decide to go on a two-week trek. While stuffing the one backpack she is allowed, Francey realizes that there is no room for her shampoo, no room for her shiatsu foot massager, and no room for fourteen vaginal DHEA suppositories that will melt while hiking since they are anticipating temperatures well into the 90's. Not to mention, discarding those plastic blister packs would be an environmental disaster. Francey, now quite the expert on vaginal dryness , decides this would be a good time to try the vagina pill that goes in her mouth.*

8

A PILL A DAY TO KEEP DRYNESS AWAY

THOUGH LOCAL VAGINAL estrogen and vaginal DHEA do a terrific job of treating thin, dry vaginal tissue, many of my patients tell me they would prefer just to take a pill. For most, it's a matter of convenience. I get it—local products require more than a few steps: You need to store the pills/inserts/rings/creams somewhere the kids won't find them, retrieve the product, bring it into the bathroom, remove your clothes, use an applicator or your fingers to apply/insert said product, and then deal with the applicator and/or packaging. Washing your reusable estrogen cream applicator in the dishwasher can present a problem if you are not the one unloading the dishwasher. Not to mention, do you really want your vaginal applicator next to your soup spoons? Popping a pill at the same time you take your vitamins and thyroid medication is a lot simpler—not to mention, it can be done in public with your clothes on.

In some instances, women are actually ashamed of the need to use something to alleviate dryness, and they don't want their partner or husband to know they are not as naturally moist and sexy as when they were twenty. The ReVIVE Survey found that eighty-one percent of women who use local vaginal estrogen have a "secret ritual" to insert or apply the product so their partner doesn't know they are using it. Ninety three percent of women however, use nothing and simply grit their teeth and endure painful sex, or go into avoidance mode.

While some would rather take a pill, others have to take a pill

While physical challenges can occur at any age, the older someone is, the more likely they are to have arthritis or other physical challenge that make it impractical or impossible to open a suppository, insert a ring or apply a vaginal cream.

If you fall into a group who, for whatever reason, would rather put a pill in your mouth than put something in your vagina, there is an option.

Ospemifene (brand name Osphena™) is a daily oral pill to alleviate vaginal dryness and painful intercourse. It was originally released in 2013 and FDA-approved for the treatment of painful sex. In 2019, the FDA expanded its approval to also cover vaginal dryness. Although widely used, it has never caught on to the same degree as the local vaginal estrogens.

UTI Relief

Aside from enabling sexual activity, ospemifene may be the answer for woman with recurrent urinary tract infections. In the pre-approval clinical trials, interestingly, and not surprisingly, urinary tract infections increased with initial use, likely due to an increase in intercourse after alleviation of painful intercourse. However, after six months of use, the rate of UTIs were dramatically reduced, equivalent to what is seen with the use of local vaginal estrogens. So, while it is not advertised by the company, and is an off label use of ospemifene, (meaning the FDA did not approve it for this purpose) this is an enormous benefit, particularly for older women who are not able or willing to put something in their vagina but can swallow a pill.

How Ospemifene Works

Ospemifene is not estrogen but is classified as a selective estrogen receptor modulator, or SERM. SERMs are drugs that either block estrogen pathways or activate estrogen pathways in specific tissues.

There are lots of other SERMS you may be familiar with:

- Clomiphene stimulates ovarian tissue and is used as a fertility drug.
- Tamoxifen blocks estrogen pathways in the breast, which is why it is useful in the prevention of breast cancer.
- Raloxifene activates estrogen pathways in bone (to treat osteopenia and osteoporosis) and also blocks estrogen pathways in the breast (to prevent breast cancer).
- Ospemifene activates estrogen pathways in vaginal and vulvar tissue and essentially has the same effect as local vaginal estrogen to alleviate painful intercourse and vaginal dryness due to menopause. It also stimulates estrogen receptors in bone (it was initially developed as a potential osteoporosis drug!) but does not work as well on bone as raloxifene.

Advantages

- Again, many women find a pill easier to take than putting something in their vagina.
- For women who would like to avoid hormones, this is an alternative.
- Ospemifene does not increase the risk of breast cancer.

- Because ospemifene appears to block estrogen receptors in breast tissue, most experts feel that it is a good option for women who have breast cancer. Having said that, it has not been tested in women with breast cancer. And although it is reassuring to know that it shrunk breast tumors in rats, women are not rats.

Disadvantages

- Between seven to nine percent of women have hot flashes when using this product. So, if you are having a hard time with flashes, this is probably not your best option.
- Many women are reluctant to take a systemic drug for a local problem.
- Ospemifene interferes with systemic estrogen. Women cannot take ospemifene if they are using a transdermal or oral systemic estrogen for relief of hot flashes.
- Women who are taking another SERM, such as tamoxifen or raloxifene, cannot take ospemifene.
- All SERMS potentially increase the risk of developing blood clots, which may precipitate a stroke or heart attack. That is why the FDA issued a warning for women with a history of blood clots who are considering taking ospemifene. In the clinical trials for ospemifene, which lasted for over a year, the incidence rates of thromboembolic stoke (caused by a blood clot) was 0.72 per thousand women. The incidence of hemorrhagic stroke was 1.45 per thousand women. In the placebo group, stroke occurred in 1.04 per thousand women. In other words, this is a theoretical concern as opposed to an actual complication that occurred in the clinical trials. Having said that, many women with a history of stroke or heart attack may choose to avoid taking any SERM.

- Ospemifene weakly stimulates the tissue that lines the uterus, and there is a concern that it may precipitate abnormal bleeding or cause changes leading to uterine cancer. However, there is no evidence of an increased risk of uterine cancer. In the clinical trials, women had regular uterine biopsies, and there was no increase in uterine cancer rates. This is reassuring, but any woman, whether she takes ospemifene or not, should evaluate any post-menopausal spotting or bleeding.
- The FDA states that women with breast cancer should not use this drug, not because it has been shown to be harmful, but because it has never been tested in women with breast cancer. However, most menopause experts consider ospemifene to be an excellent estrogen alternative because breast tissue is not stimulated. ▼

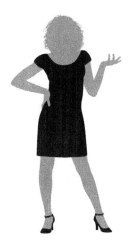

❯ *DEVASTATING NEWS: Francey's beloved 98-year-old grandmother Fern not so unexpectedly dies. The blow is softened by the unexpected bequeath to Francey of her entire estate, which is far larger than anyone imagined given that her life savings was in a Folger's coffee tin hidden under her bed. Francey immediately quits her job, books a trip to Paris, breaks up with Randy (nice but prefers tents to five-star hotels), and decides the time is right to laser her face, laser off that ridiculous tattoo she got when she got divorced, and, of course, laser her vagina.*

WHY MONA LISA IS SMILING

THE CO_2 LASER has been available for years as a method to treat myriad skin conditions: the removal of excessive or unwanted hair, wrinkle reduction, and tattoo removal. And since 2014, the CO_2 laser has been FDA-cleared for use on vaginal tissue.

Medical studies prove that the CO_2 laser, like the other prescription products already discussed, increases vaginal lubrication and elasticity and reduces or eliminates pain during sexual activity. But buyer beware: Though many dermatologists and plastic surgeons offer to laser and "rejuvenate" your genitals, this is a procedure that is best done by an expert.

Laser Treatment Is Not Vaginal Rejuvenation!

I do not use and have never used the term "vaginal rejuvenation." "Vaginal rejuvenation" is a marketing not a medical term and has no precise definition. Genitourinary syndrome of menopause is a medical condition, and like other medical conditions, it is defined by very specific physical changes and symptoms for which there are recognized treatment options.

I am aware that some companies and doctors market treatments, including lasers, to "improve" the appearance of or shrink the vagina. The CO_2 laser is a medical device and should not be used for cosmetic purposes.

Why Would a Woman Choose to Laser Her Vagina?

Despite the many safe options to treat vaginal dryness and painful sex, only seven percent of affected women use a prescription product that goes beyond what a lubricant can do. The number of women treated for these symptoms is even lower in survivors of a gynecologic or breast cancer.

There are a variety of reasons that this number is so low:

1. Many women are not bothered by the inability to have intercourse; they think it's not important enough to treat.
2. Some women don't want to use a product on a regular basis.
3. Many women, despite reassurances, are concerned about side effects from a prescription option such as a local vaginal estrogen, ospemifene, or DHEA.
4. Often a woman's physician advises against using local vaginal estrogen.

If you fall into the first category, you are definitely not even reading this. But the other categories are a different story, and too many women either abandon sexual activity altogether or put up with the pain.

For women in categories two through four, the CO_2 laser is an alternative solution.

How Laser Treatments Work

You know from reading chapter 1 that the top layer of healthy, estrogenized vaginal tissue has abundant collagen and fibrin and a rich blood supply. Post-menopause, the top layer is pretty much nonexistent.

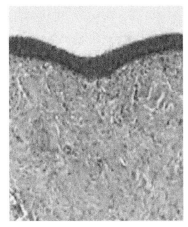 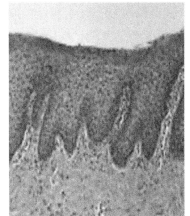

PRE-LASER   POST-LASER

Carbon dioxide (CO_2) lasers deliver controlled energy to stimulate your own cells to make more collagen and fibrin and increase blood supply. The post laser vaginal wall is indistinguishable from a pre-menopausal vaginal wall.

Mona Lisa Touch™ is the brand name of the most commonly used CO_2 laser. There are many others, but the device I use is Mona Lisa Touch™ because it is the brand that was used in the majority of published scientific trials.

The result of laser treatment is the restoration of lubrication and elasticity that has vanished as a consequence of menopause. One of the major advantages of laser treatments (other than the convenience of not having to do something on a regular basis) is that the laser is used not only to treat the entire vaginal canal but also the tissues at the opening of the vagina and on the vulva as well. Hence, Mona Lisa is smiling because her vagina is good to go.

Like the prescription options, the laser treats other symptoms of genitourinary syndrome of menopause, including vulvar itching, urinary urgency, and painful intercourse. Early data suggests that the laser may also help reduce or eliminate recurrent urinary tract infections.

In clinical trials—and my experience—approximately ninety-five percent of women report that after the treatment they have significantly less dryness, pain, and irritation, along with a dramatic improvement in sexual pleasure. Vaginal laser treatment has been used both here and in Europe in hundreds of thousands of women. No substantiated, significant safety issues or adverse reactions have been reported.

What to Expect

Laser treatment involves three five-minute sessions performed in a doctor's office, spaced six weeks apart. It is critical to have an evaluation prior to signing up to ensure that you will benefit. Once it is confirmed that your symptoms are a result of vaginal atrophy as a consequence of genitourinary syndrome of menopause, you are good to go.

After assuming your favorite gynecologic position (who invented stirrups anyway?), a local anesthesia cream is applied to the vaginal opening and vulva. Occasionally, some women will feel a slight burning from the cream, but it takes only a few minutes for numbness to set in. (Many of my patients inquire about getting a prescription for this anesthetic cream for their next bikini wax ... just saying.)

The cream is then wiped off, and a slender wand is placed in the vagina. I then treat roughly sixty spots in the vagina by withdrawing and rotating the wand. The laser settings ensure that by using this technique, the entire surface of the vagina is treated. This goes faster than you think with someone who is experienced. My patients report feeling only gentle vibration while the laser is in the vagina.

If you smell something burning, it is not you! Residual anesthetic cream causes a burning odor when it is hit by

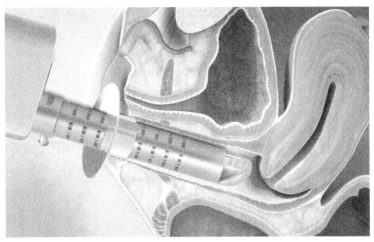

The vaginal laser wand placed in the vagina.

the laser beam, so don't panic.

After the vagina is treated, I switch to a different laser head with a small, flat surface to treat the vestibule and, if needed, any dry areas outside of the vestibule.

The whole thing takes less than ten minutes, and there will be no pain. Promise.

Afterward, most women are totally fine other than being aware that "something was done." I have the occasional patient that does feel slightly uncomfortable, but it rarely lasts more than a day. Slathering the vulva with Aquaphor™ for the first twenty-four hours is helpful, particularly because it protects the area from urine, which tends to burn when it hits it. Most women go about their business other than the business of intercourse. Refrain for at least two or three days.

How Soon Does It Work?

This is highly variable. There is a big difference between the woman who, prior to the laser, was having intercourse on a regular basis but just wants to stop using her local estrogen and the woman who has not had intercourse in twenty years. Some women tell me they are aware of a big difference after the first treatment, but most need all three treatments to get where they need to go. Occasionally, I need to do a fourth treatment. And just like women who are not pain-free after a prescription product, many women, post-laser, need pelvic floor physical therapy to get tight, painful pelvic muscles to relax. (The next chapter deals with that issue!)

How Long Does It Last?

The results generally last around a year, which means that an annual booster treatment is required to maintain the results. Having said that, I have patients who need a booster after ten months and others who can go fourteen to sixteen months. Your vagina did not read the manufacturer's manual, and there is a huge difference in degree of dryness, usage, and response!

The Downside of Laser Treatments

The main problem is that medical CO_2 laser treatments for vaginal dryness are expensive and not covered by insurance. One woman told me the choice was between pleasurable sex for a year and a vacation in Florida for a week. She chose sex for a year. Prices do vary widely, but sometimes the lowest price is offered by someone with the lowest level of experience. It is important to make sure that whoever is doing your treatment not only does a careful evaluation prior to the procedure but also routinely treats both the vagina and the vestibule.

Warning!

And whatever you do, do not have this procedure per-

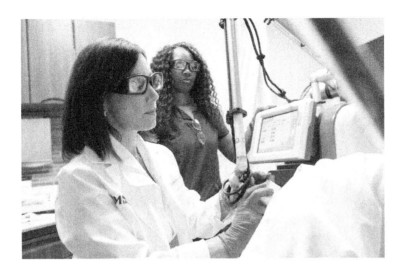

formed by a plastic surgeon or a dermatologist! Think about it: Would you have your gynecologist do your face-lift? Although it is not a difficult procedure to perform, only gynecologists have the expertise to evaluate the vaginal and vulvar tissue and determine the cause of your pain (sometimes pain during intercourse has nothing to do with vaginal dryness and will not be helped by a laser treatment), and routinely perform vaginal procedures. Often non-gynecologists treat the vaginal canal but not the opening or external tissues. So tell your plastic surgeon to stick to your wrinkly face and leave it to your gynecologist to restore wrinkles to your vaginal walls!

A Cautionary Tale

I met a woman when I was speaking at a cancer survivor event who, prior to her cancer diagnosis, suffered from terrible pain during sex. Her plastic surgeon, assuming her problem was dryness, offered to treat her using a vaginal laser. The first round did not help, so she went back for an additional two treatments. Thousands of dollars and months later, she finally went to a gynecologist, who diagnosed ovarian cancer as the root of her pain.

Advantages
- You do not need to do anything on a regular basis.
- There is no messiness or ongoing need to put something in the vagina.
- Both the vagina and the vestibule are treated.
- It's ideal for women with breast cancer who are reluctant to or have been advised against using hormonal treatments.

Disadvantages
- Treatment requires three office visits, which takes time and may be inconvenient.
- The results generally last only around a year, which means that an annual booster treatment is required.
- The laser is not covered by insurance
- The procedure is not available everywhere.

FAQ About CO2 Laser Therapy
Is radiofrequency the same thing as the laser?

CO_2 laser therapy is not the same thing as radiofrequency, a completely different treatment that often claims to help genitourinary syndrome of menopause, even though there has been no research to confirm that is the case.

Can the laser penetrate too deep and injure my internal organs?

The depth of penetration is roughly 0.03 mm to 0.05 mm, which translates to less than the depth of a credit card. So, no, it is impossible for the laser to penetrate beyond the vaginal wall.

I have lichen sclerosus. Can I still get laser treatment?

Yes, you can treat vaginal atrophy with the laser even if you also have lichen sclerosus. Some doctors say that the laser will help treat lichen sclerosis, but currently, the science does not bear that out, so you will need to continue using your topical steroids. Having said that, I have had many patients who have had improvement in cracking or splitting of their skin.

Does the laser help with skin changes from radiation treatments?

There has been essentially no research done in women who have dry, painful skin after undergoing pelvic radiation for treatment of cancer. Though there is no reason to believe it will be harmful, the fibrotic changes that occur post-radiation may not respond to stimulation with the laser.

I have read about complications such as scarring and burning. How often do those happen?

In the clinical trials, when women are closely monitored and the laser is done correctly, there are no reports of burning or scarring. Although you do see those claims online, none of them have been substantiated, which would require documenting an exam prior to the treatment followed by documenting an exam after it. Complications are always possible with any procedure, but the design of the laser, and the safety mechanisms in place, make these kinds of events unlikely. Keep in mind, this same laser has been used for a very long time on a variety of skin conditions, including for wrinkle removal and tattoo removal. ▼

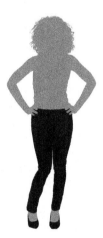

> *AT FRANCEY'S FAREWELL party, her cousin Linda is clearly furious that Grandma did not leave her anything—and furious that her nemesis Francey not only has had an enviable string of hot boyfriends, but also evidently has the vagina of a thirty-year-old. After her second martini, Linda blurts out that she hates Francey, has always hated Francey, and, by the way, despite using a bucketful of lube and trying every estrogen product on the market, her vagina is like a Venus fly trap. After her third martini, she throws her arms around Francey, and admits that she doesn't actually hate her, she is just really frustrated.*

10

OTHER BARRIERS TO ENTRY

YOU'VE DONE IT all: tried the lubricants, moisturizers, and every prescription product on the market and even shelled out for laser treatment. But there is still no way, no how that penis is going in there without your neighbors calling 911 because of the screams. Before you throw in the towel and decide celibacy is inevitable, read on.

Many treatment "failures" have happened because the wrong thing was being treated. Everything I talk about in this book is specifically to treat the tissue changes that occur as a result of low estrogen. There is a long list of other medical conditions that cause painful or impossible intercourse. (My book Sex Rx gets into those details.)

In many cases, the product you are using ensures that the vagina is treated, but the vestibule is not. It bears repeating: It doesn't matter how nice the room is if you can't get through the door.

Even if your problem were due to menopause, estrogen, DHEA, ospemifene, and laser only treat tissue. They do not

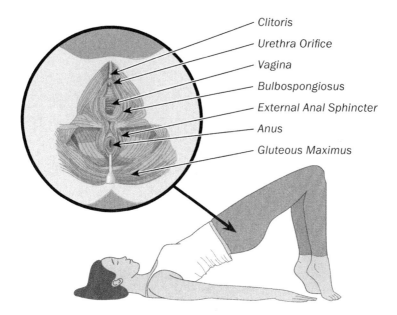

Clitoris
Urethra Orifice
Vagina
Bulbospongiosus
External Anal Sphincter
Anus
Gluteous Maximus

treat the underlying pelvic floor muscles, a critical component of pain-free intercourse. Meet your pelvic floor.

Hello, Pelvic Floor

The pelvic floor is made up of multiple muscle groups that support and surround all the good stuff—your clitoris, vagina, bladder, and bowels.

These muscle groups function as a strong trampoline that supports not only the bladder, but also the uterus and the rectum. When all the muscles work together, the "trampoline" is able to contract and relax in a coordinated fashion.

Pelvic floor muscles are responsible for bladder control, bowel control, and vagina control. When it comes to pain-free intercourse, the ability of the muscles to relax is the important part.

Your Vagina Isn't Stupid

Normally, when a woman becomes aroused, her body

prepares to let a penis in, the biological purpose of sex. In preparation, the pelvic floor muscles relax, causing the vagina to lengthen and expand. The muscles around the opening of the vagina also relax, which is the vagina's way of saying, "I'm ready—come on in."

But if your past sexual attempts resulted in pain, your vagina goes into "Are you kidding? You are not coming in here just to cause me more pain" mode. Your pelvic muscles will involuntarily contract in an attempt to keep the penis out.

It's actually not unusual for dry, thin tissues to have been successfully treated yet there is still pain with intercourse. Your vagina isn't stupid: It has spent years developing these protective mechanisms. Your muscle memory does not know that your vaginal tissues are now well lubricated and whatever originally caused the pain has been eliminated. Your vagina, in fact your entire pelvis, has been in protective, "keep out" mode for so long that the pelvic and vaginal muscles will continue to contract involuntarily in an attempt to keep out a penis that could potentially cause pain. Muscles that are contracted not only keep the penis out, which at its extreme is a condition known as vaginismus, but are also really painful. So you need to treat the vaginal tissue as well as the muscles that support and surround the vagina.

And that is where pelvic floor physical therapy comes in.

A Personal Trainer for Your Pelvis

I've heard it a million times. When discussing solutions for vaginal dryness, my patients expect me to bring up lubricants, moisturizers, medications. It's when I introduce the topic of pelvic floor physical therapy that I get reactions like:

"You're kidding, right?"

"She's not going to put her hands in there!" (This is accompanied by a horrified look.)

"Do I really need that? Can't you just give me a different medicine?"

Well, no, I'm not kidding. Yes, she is going to put her hands in there. Yes, you do need that, and no, I can't just give you a different medicine.

Consider if you broke your leg. Once the cast comes off, working with a physical therapist would be a standard part of rehabilitation and the restoration of normal function. After a break or serious injury, your muscles don't function properly as a result of trauma and disuse.

The same goes for the muscles that support your pelvic organs. If your vagina or pelvis has been traumatized by painful sex, physical therapy is a key component of your recovery.

Pelvic floor physical therapists have done additional, very specialized training in the treatment of pelvic disorders, including gynecologic, urologic, muscular, and neurologic problems. Many women are skeptical when advised to seek the help of a physical therapist. These same women usually become the greatest advocates of the treatment. As a gynecologist, I can almost always fix the problem that initially caused the pain, but the PT is the only person who can erase the muscle memory, eliminate pelvic floor muscle tension, strengthen atrophied muscles, and restore normal, healthy functioning. In my practice, I rely so much on my team of pelvic physical therapists that I refer to them as my "magicians."

Painful intercourse is not the only ailment pelvic floor physical therapists treat. The list also includes urinary incontinence, fecal (bowel) incontinence, constipation, pelvic pain from endometriosis or other conditions, interstitial cystitis, vulvodynia, and even lower back pain.

In addition, women who experience urinary urgency and frequency due to genitourinary syndrome of menopause also benefit from pelvic floor PT to help calm down those overactive bladder muscles!

Working With a Pelvic Floor Physical Therapist

Because it is a mystery to most women what a pelvic floor physical therapist does, it helps to know what to expect when signing up. Her office will look like a gynecologist's office but without the stirrups. She'll start by taking a detailed history, not only about your sexual issues, but also your general health, with a particular focus on bowel and bladder problems seeing as constipation and incontinence go hand in hand with pelvic floor muscles that are not properly functioning.

In the first part of the physical exam, the PT will evaluate things like your posture, abdominal strength, and general physical fitness. The pelvic exam will be kind of like a gynecologic exam without the speculum; however, it's likely to include a number of elements that will be unfamiliar to you. It'll start with a thorough visual evaluation of the vulvar skin and vestibule. The PT will use a cotton swab to touch each zone to see which areas are painful. She'll then gently introduce a gloved, lubricated finger into the vagina in order to systematically touch specific muscle groups that make up the pelvic floor. By gently applying pressure to various pelvic floor muscle groups, the therapist will determine whether the problem is due to tight muscles, known as a hypertonic pelvic floor. She'll feel for inappropriate knots, contractions, and inflammation of the muscles and the connective tissue. She may identify a specific, isolated, tender spot, known as a trigger point, that when touched reproduces the pain felt during intercourse.

The physical therapist also will evaluate your overall muscle strength and coordination by asking you to squeeze her finger using your pelvic muscles. This is similar to the maneuver you do when performing a Kegel exercise.

The experienced pelvic floor physical therapist will not only treat the problem, but also play an important role in helping your physician determine the source of the problem in the first place. In performing a thorough musculoskeletal evaluation of the pelvis, spine, and hips, she'll often find pelvic asymmetry and muscle imbalances in women with pelvic and sexual pain. Often the location of the pain is not where the pelvic pain originates. For example, tight hip flexor muscles tilt the pelvis and cause tension in the pelvic floor muscles, which, in turn, contributes to pelvic pain and dysfunction.

Once the source of the pain is identified, the therapist will use a number of modalities for treatment, including techniques such as myofascial (tissue) release and joint mobilization. Muscle spasms will be eliminated using manual soft tissue work and trigger point release directly on the pelvic floor muscles through the vagina and occasionally the rectum. (This is definitely a hands-on treatment!)

Your PT may also use biofeedback, which involves placing electrodes either externally or internally to register the electrical activity of muscles. The information, displayed on a monitor while your muscle activity is occurring, shows when your actions are causing muscles to tighten or relax.

Because muscles that remain tense and contracted at all times cause pain, one of the major goals of biofeedback is to reteach them to relax completely when they are not needed and learn to recruit others in a coordinated fashion when they are. Ultimately, you learn to control your muscles without the feedback. These techniques really work to eliminate pain, improve tissue integrity via increased circulation and oxygenation, and restore normal resting muscle tone and length.

If your case is severe, your physician or physical therapist may augment therapy with strategies to relax your tight muscles, such as diazepam suppositories (Valium™ for your vagina!), trigger point injections with local anesthetic, or Botox™ injections.

Ultimately, pelvic floor physical therapy allows a woman to improve function and also allows her to engage in intercourse without the vaginal and pelvic floor muscles painfully and inappropriately contracting.

Finding a Pelvic Floor Physical Therapist

Unlike dentists and hairdressers, you generally can't just ask a savvy girlfriend who her pelvic floor physical therapist is and go with her recommendation. If your gynecologist works with a PT, he or she will make a referral. Most major medical centers have a large PT department, including pelvic PT.

But beware: Just as even good gynecologists don't always know much about treating vaginal dryness, a PT who says she does pelvic work isn't necessarily an expert. Ideally you want to go to someone who does pelvic floor PT exclusively as opposed to someone who treats knees on Mondays, hips on Tuesdays, and vaginas every other Wednesday. When you call to make an appointment, ask, "What percentage of your practice is devoted to pelvic floor physical therapy?" If the response is less than fifty percent, you may want to keep looking. A good starting point is to go to www.pelvicrehab.com, a national website exclusively devoted to pelvic floor therapists who have completed a specific course of training. For a more extensive list, go to the American Physical Therapy Association's website, www.womenshealthapta.org.

Some women do not have an experienced pelvic therapist in their area or do not have insurance that will cover the cost of the sessions. If you need pelvic floor therapy but have no access, or are a DIY kind of woman, you can start with at-home dilator therapy.

Vaginal Dilator Therapy

When someone comes to my office, the first clue that they are not in Kansas anymore is the set of multicolored dildoes sitting prominently on my counter.

I often use these dilators to evaluate the elasticity of a patient's vagina to see what she is able to tolerate prior to treatment, and then to assess how she is progressing. Most penises are the size of my orange, purple, or blue dilator. For obvious reasons, I learned a long time ago never to ask what size dilator a male partner is if he is in the room.

Vaginal dilator therapy has three purposes:

Dilators get the vagina used to having something inside of it. Even if the tissue is well lubricated and stretchy, a history of painful sex initiates a cycle of pain–fear–muscle spasms–more pain that results in the vagina constricting at any attempt to have intercourse. By starting small and then increasing gradually to whatever penis size is in your life, the vaginal tissues "learn" to accommodate having something inside without a pain response being triggered.

Graduated dilators also gradually stretch tissues that are tight and have lost their elasticity, which is often the case if a woman has vaginal atrophy from hormonal changes or a skin condition or her vagina has been shortened by radiation or surgery.

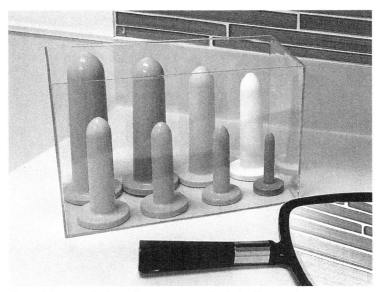

Something you don't see in every gynecologist's office.

The other important advantage to using a dilator is that you will know when you are ready for intercourse. That way, when you have sex with an actual penis, your pelvis won't panic.

Where Do You Get Dilators?

My go-to for medical-grade, consumer-friendly, color-coded vaginal dilators is Soul Source™ (soulsource.com). Graduated dilators can be purchased individually but generally come in sets of four to eight, ranging from 1⁄2 inch to 1-5⁄8 inches in diameter. I know what you are thinking.

What is the diameter of an "average" erect penis?

The average diameter of an erect penis is 1.5 inches (3.8 centimeters), so if you can get the 1-5⁄8-inch dilator in comfortably, you are good to go. If you want to know the

95

diameter of your partner's penis, use a piece of string or ribbon to take a measurement. (I will leave you to come up with the creative response as to why you are putting a ribbon around his erect penis.) Tell him his result in centimeters, not inches, because that always sounds much bigger. No matter what the measurement is, look impressed. Never use the word "average" when announcing a man's penis diameter.

"Alternative" Dilators

Although it's tempting to use phallic-shaped items from your kitchen (celery, zucchini, bananas, cucumbers) or candles (birthday, Hanukkah, tapers, pillars), I don't recommend it. Ask any ER doc who has removed one of those objects from a mortified patient. If you must, put a condom over it in case of breakage!

How to Use Your Graduated Dilator

Once you own a dilator, what do you do with it? Unless your tissue is already in good shape, put it away. Unlike the new shoes that you can't wait to wear, you need to be patient. A dilator is rarely the first step in eliminating pain from vaginal dryness. First you treat the tissue, then you treat the muscle. Can you do both simultaneously? Yes, but only if you are able to get a small dilator in without pain.

Once you get the go-ahead, here's what to do:

Step 1: If possible, start with a warm bath (to relax you and your pelvic floor muscles), and make sure you have at least fifteen minutes of privacy. Putting a dildo in your vagina if your teenage son is about to burst into your room is not going to work.

Step 2: Lie in bed on your back with your knees bent and slightly apart. This is not yoga class. Be comfortable! Use pillows to support your head and back.

Step 3: Apply a generous amount of lubrication to the opening of your vagina and to the tip of the smallest dilator. If the dilator is silicone, be sure to use a water-based lubricant.

Step 4: Bear down slightly, and gently slide the dilator in as far as it will go.

Step 5: If there is no pain or resistance, continue to insert larger dilators. The dilator that should be used to initiate your therapy is the largest dilator that does not cause any pain with insertion. At some point you will start to feel resistance, discomfort, or burning. Stop. Don't push it. This is not the gym, and you don't need to use the heaviest weight. You will get there eventually.

Step 6: Leave the largest dilator that does not cause pain in place for at least five minutes. Concentrate on letting your vaginal tissues relax around it. Your buttocks and thighs should be relaxed as well. Don't forget to breathe. A little Mozart is not a bad idea.

Step 7: Repeat steps 1 through 6 on a daily basis, if possible. It's OK if you miss a day.

Step 8: When you are at the point where the biggest dilator you have been using slides in without resistance or discomfort, it is time to go up to the next size. This can take days or weeks.

Step 9: When you are ready to go up to the next size, continue to use the smaller dilator to start your session for at least a few days before you insert the next size.

Wash your dilators with antibacterial soap and water and dry them well before you put them away. Store them in a box labeled "2018 tax returns" so your teenage daughter will not find them when she is raiding your drawers to borrow some tights.

When first using a dilator, light spotting is not unusual, but you should never experience severe pain or heavy bleeding. If you do, or if you are unable to comfortably insert a dilator, see your doctor before proceeding.

Sometimes it is necessary to coat the dilator with local anesthetic jelly (you will need a prescription for this). In other cases, a muscle relaxant is useful (Valium™ for your vagina!). Once you can comfortably put something in your vagina that is slightly larger than your partner's penis, you are ready for the real thing.

Which brings me to the next point: When dealing with any kind of pain associated with intercourse, sometimes you are better off avoiding an actual penis until the problem has been solved. Severe, longstanding cases of painful attempts at intercourse will cause your pelvis to panic and your vagina to contract as a protective mechanism. So pelvic floor physical therapy and/or vaginal dilators may be needed to teach your vagina that putting something in it will not be painful.

I typically tell women who have been having painful intercourse to stop trying until the problem has been eliminated. When I tell my patients intercourse is temporarily off the table, most women are relieved to have "permission" to stop. I am very specific that I am not saying to stop having sex, just to stop trying to have vaginal penetration.

Bad joke:
Woman to her husband: *"My gynecologist says I can't have intercourse for two weeks."*
Husband: *"What does your dentist say?"*

Other Barriers to Entry

Slip Sliding Away does not address relationship, past history of trauma, or other psychological barriers that impact on the ability to have pain free sexual activity. This is an example of the role of a trained sex therapist who is trauma informed. See chapter 12 for more about sex therapy.

In addition, I again need to emphasize that there are many other vulvar, vaginal, and pelvic conditions besides genitourinary syndrome of menopause that sabotage the ability to have pain free, pleasurable sex. While the details are in my book Sex Rx, it is critical to be evaluated by an expert in vulvar and vaginal conditions.

Financial Barriers to Entry

A few years ago, I was sitting across from Jill, a long-term patient of mine, who had come in for her annual exam. During her previous visit, we had spent a lot of time talking about strategies to deal with painful intercourse, which had left her pretty much in avoidance mode. She had left my office that day with a prescription for a local vaginal estrogen along with a number of over-the-counter product recommendations.

"So how are things going sexually?" I asked. She gave a dismissive wave of her hand, and said, "We gave up on that."

I asked what happened with the products we'd discussed the last time.

"Frankly," she said, "between my husband's issues and my issues, we added it up and realized we couldn't afford it. It's OK."

Can't afford sex? Sex is one of the few pleasures in life that's free! That's like saying you can't afford to go for a walk or to give your partner a nice massage. Shame on me. Up until that point, I had never really considered the cost of the products that, for some people, don't just makes intercourse pleasurable—they make it possible. Even if you have insurance that covers part or all of the cost of the prescription products, many Americans are uninsured or underinsured. Over-the-counter products are rarely covered.

I added it up and was shocked at the economics of post-menopause sex. Here are the potential annual costs for a couple who has sex twice a week:

Silicone lubricant ....$60 to $120
Local vaginal estrogen .... About $2,500
(The price varies widely depending on the product)
Long-acting vaginal moisturizer $240
Erectile dysfunction medication........................ $3,000
Vaginal laser .... $1,500 to $3,000
Doctor's visits to get prescriptions $300

Not everyone requires all of these products, but depending on what someone needs, it's dramatically cheaper to go to the movies once a week than to make love. And that's not including the cost of new lingerie, candles, a vibrator, and maybe the occasional bottle of champagne. I wondered how many of my patients had given up their sex lives not just because it was difficult or painful, but also because if they had to choose between buying groceries and buying Viagra™, eating trumped pleasure.

In 2018, I was interviewed by The New York Times for a piece about the high price of drugs to treat sexual health and the fact that those products are rarely covered by insurance.

As stated in the Times, "While women privately fume about the costs, drug makers have been able to raise their prices without a public outcry in part because the topic—

women's sex lives and their vaginas—is still pretty much taboo."

One of the high points of my life was when I woke up the morning after the article ran and saw that one of my quotes was on the front page of the paper as "the quote of the day"!

> 66 *Unlike EpiPen, women are not going to be rising up and saying,* 'My vagina is dry and I don't want to pay 2,000 to 3,000 dollars a year,'" *said Dr. Lauren Streicher, the medical director of the Northwestern Medicine Center for Sexual Medicine and Menopause.* 99
>
> —The New York Times, 6/03/18

Cutting Your Costs

You can get some breaks by checking out the coupons on pharmaceutical websites. See if your insurance plan will cover the over-the-counter products if you have a prescription. Ask your doctor if vaginal estrogen once a week rather than twice a week will do the trick. Sometimes a less convenient but equally effective product will be covered. Check out meds from other developed countries such as Canada and Mexico or from European nations, but stay away from those manufactured by developing countries.

Finally, tell your children that next Mother's Day, skip the flowers and send some lube. ▼

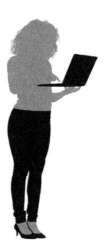

>*FRANCEY, BEING CHARITABLE and quite the dry vagina expert, recommends that Linda see her doctor to figure out why Linda is still having pain despite using estrogen. Francey's doctor, sadly, now has a three-month wait. In the meantime, in addition to calling every day and asking if there are cancellations, Linda decides to consult Dr. Google. In the midst of a 3:00 a.m. search, she becomes convinced that her problem is not dryness from menopause but vulvar cancer.*

CALLING DR. GOOGLE

I GET IT. Why take off work, sit in someone's waiting room, pay a fee, and have a potentially painful and/or humiliating exam just to get a diagnosis you can get in the privacy of your own home, fully dressed, at any hour, from a source that does not require stirrups, speculums, or insurance?

According to the Pew Research Center, eighty percent of internet users consult it for pretty much everything that ails them in lieu of seeing a doctor. There are 40,000 health-related searches on Google every second, which translates to over 3.5 billion health searches per day.

Here's the Problem

When you (or someone you know) has received a diagnosis or has a symptom and are looking for information, the internet can be a good thing. On the other hand, the information could be misleading, wrong, and/or terrifying.

Google HPV (a very common search term) and you will learn that human papilloma virus is responsible for cervical, anal, vulvar, lung, and throat cancer. All terrifyingly true, but the majority of women with a diagnosis of HPV on their Pap test need no treatment. In most cases, the body clears the virus, and a follow-up Pap is all that is required. The overwhelming majority of women do not get cancer.

But human nature being what it is, most women will assume the worst, panic, become anxious, and, in many cases, with the tap of a link, buy one of the many worthless "miracle cures" that just happen to pop up on the same site that answers your questions about HPV.

Be Your Own Doctor!

Self-diagnosis based on an internet search of symptoms is also dangerous. Studies have shown that only thirty-five percent of adults follow up with a physician. Most assume they have something more serious than they actually have.

Eighty percent of adults Google their symptoms before a doctor or emergency department visit. One study that surveyed adults in an ER found that almost all had looked up their symptoms and arrived having "self-diagnosed" their condition. Only twenty-nine percent left the emergency department with their perceived diagnosis confirmed.

What's Good About Using the Internet for Health Info

In some cases, checking out symptoms online will get someone to a doctor. Good information can also keep someone from going to a doctor unnecessarily.

And, yes, an informed patient is a really good thing. It makes my job much easier when I have a patient who has done her "homework" and knows a lot about her condition. The key is, she needs access to scientifically accurate information.

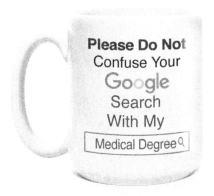

Getting Good Information

A lot of folks assume that if they are on a medical website, like WebMD, they are getting accurate information. Sometimes that is the case, but you can't count on it. Every once in a while, I do a search on WebMD and am horrified by the lack of information, the misinformation, or the out-of-date information.

Whether you are checking out symptoms to see if your headache is eyestrain or brain cancer or looking for potential side effects before you pop a pill, it would be nice to have some reassurance that the information you are reading is medically accurate.

Tips to Know If a Site is Medically Accurate
- Look at who wrote the article. A twenty-five-year-old freelance writer is not the best person to get information from on local vaginal estrogen, even if she supposedly interviewed experts. I have seen my own quotes taken out of context many times.
- If an expert didn't write it, did an expert review it? And is the "expert" really an expert? An MD after a name is

not always a guarantee that he or she is an expert in that area.

- When was it written? Many sites avoid putting dates on their articles, and you have no way of knowing how current the information is.
- Is the site sponsored? If someone is trying to sell you something, beware.

My List of Trustworthy Websites

Although I recommend these websites as having information that is generally up to date and accurate, my endorsement doesn't mean I agree with everything on them (except for my own website, of course!). Chapter 14 has a complete list of resources.

DrStreicher.com

I wrote every word that appears on my site, and every article has been exhaustively researched. My site has articles on virtually every aspect of women's health. My favorite section includes my articles on the history of medicine. Though I do update, there may be the occasional article that needs refreshing.

UpToDate.Com

This go-to site for physicians and other health care professionals requires a paid subscription, but there is also has a free patient portal. All articles were written not only by physicians, but by a top expert in that field. There are comprehensive articles on virtually every medical condition, including pediatrics. The information in the patient portal is understandable and, though written for consumers, not dumbed down. And the reason it is called UpToDate is that every article is reviewed and updated with new information every few months. In addition, there are links to relevant sites or articles for people who want more information.

Mayo Clinic: www.mayohealth.org

This site is good for general medical information about specific symptoms, tests, and procedures. It is particularly useful when checking out a medication. There is information on both prescription and over-the-counter medications, including what a drug is made of, what it does, precautions, and its side effects.

**The National Center for Complementary
and Integrative Medicine: www.nccih.nih.gov**

Instead of relying on the "expert" at the corner health food store, go to the National Center for Complementary and Integrative Medicine's website to find accurate, up-to-date safety and efficacy information on specific herbs, supplements, and practices (such as acupuncture). You can also look up specific conditions to learn alternative and complementary options.

**The North America Menopause Society:
www.menopause.org**

The North America Menopause Society's website is intended for health care clinicians, but it has loads of consumer information on menopause. More important, it is the place to go to find a certified menopause practitioner.

**Pub Med:
www.ncbi.nlm.nih.gov/pubmed**

And for those who really want to do a deep dive, head on over to PubMed to delve into medical journals. Some require a subscription, but you can usually get a summary of the information.

Promises, Promises:
A Word About Over-the-Counter Products

Scroll the web and you're likely to be bombarded by ads for a plethora of products that promise to remove wrinkles, tighten your vagina, cure incontinence, or ensure orgasmic ecstasy. It's a wonder that anyone has anything but perfect skin, a failproof bladder, and a fabulous sex life—at least if you believe the testimonials that accompany these ads.

But in truth, most of these products haven't gone through any kind of testing process to ensure that their claims actually happen.

"How can that be," you ask, *"when virtually all of these devices and products have a U.S. Food and Drug Administration seal?"*

The answer is: An FDA-listed product doesn't equal an FDA-approved product. Despite the reassuring blue FDA logo, most over-the-counter products and devices are not FDA approved. They're simply cleared, listed, or registered by the FDA.

An FDA-approved drug goes through an extensive vetting process that not only ensures that it is safe, but also that it actually does what it says it will do. Prescription drugs are all FDA approved.

An FDA-cleared drug is a product that is sold over the counter. FDA-cleared drugs do not claim to cure a specific condition. As an example, a lubricant cannot say that it is used to treat genitourinary syndrome of menopause (a medical condition), but it can claim to "enhance intimacy." An FDA-cleared product does not go through the same approval process as an FDA-approved drug, and though it is likely to be safe, it may not necessarily do what it claims to do. In fact, most claims are simply an impressive triumph of marketing over science.

In the case of FDA-registered products, the company that makes a product, and its marketers, determine what language is used and, yes, what the product claims to do. No scientific studies are required, and no scientific studies are performed, because it's not in a company's best interest to do so. Why would a company spend millions of dollars on a study that might prove that its face cream doesn't actually eliminate wrinkles?

Similarly, the FDA doesn't regulate vitamins, herbs, or other dietary supplements, which is why so many of them claim to simply "promote" health as opposed to treating a specific illness. ▼

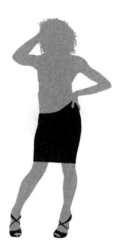

> *LINDA, CONVINCED SHE has vulvar cancer and quite sure that she needs an emergency radical vulvectomy, has decided she is not going to wait to see Francey's doctor and goes on the hunt for another doctor who knows what she is doing, takes her insurance, and can see her before her vagina falls off.*
>
> *After perusing the North American Menopause Society site, Linda finds a new gynecologist who assures her that she does not have vulvar cancer but rather severe genitourinary syndrome of menopause, along with pelvic floor muscle tension. She leaves the office with a prescription for a compounded estrogen/testosterone cream, a referral for pelvic floor physical therapy, and an appointment with a certified sex therapist who will help her deal with the fact that she subconsciously sabotages every potential relationship as a way to avoid having sex.*

12

FINDING YOUR VAGINA TEAM

ONCE YOU DO make an appointment to see a doctor, how do you know that he or she can actually help you? I hear every day from women that when they went to their doctor with their dry-giney woes, they were told, "Buy a lube." End of story.

How is it that you're such an expert, but your doctor may not be? I hate to say this, but an MD after a name is no assurance that the person to whom you are about to bare your soul—and your vagina—is an expert in your particular problem. Now that you are an expert on genitourinary syndrome of menopause, along with a menu of solutions for your dry vagina, how do you find a health care practitioner who is not only familiar with this world, but who also can help you navigate your way through menopause?

Sometimes the savvy consumer has to do a little legwork to find a clinician who is a real expert on menopausal women. A menopause expert is not necessarily your gynecologist—or a gynecologist period. An expert is a medical professional who has an interest in this area and is informed about the diagnosis and treatment of the conditions that affect women who are short on estrogen. So a menopause expert might be your gynecologist, or an internist, or a family practice doctor. It's also possible that the best clinician to help you with your particular issue may not even be a doctor, but rather an advanced practice clinician.

I want to provide you with a quick and easy-to-understand guide to what you should look for to deal with your specific issues. If you understand whom you are looking for, what kind of training is necessary for specific titles, how qualified a physician is, and how non-MD clinicians fit into the picture, you will have a better chance of getting the right treatment.

"Doctor": What's in a Title?

A "doctor" is anyone who has a doctorate-level degree. Anyone with "doctor" in front of his or her name might be a physician but might also be a dentist, podiatrist, psychologist, or English professor. If you are looking for a physician, look for an MD.

MD stands for "medical doctor." Anyone who has graduated from medical school is allowed to put MD after his or her name. Forever. DO stands for "doctor of osteopathy." An osteopath's training is essentially identical to an MD's and should be considered equivalent.

Licensing

A licensed physician is a physician who is allowed to practice medicine. Each state has its own criteria for granting licenses, but in general, licensure to practice medicine requires only proof of graduation from medical school, at least a year of clinical training, and passage of a qualifying exam. To verify that a physician is licensed, go to the Federation of State Medical Boards' website (fsmb. org). Please note that licensure is not the same thing as board certification and does not guarantee expertise in a specific field.

Board Certification

Board certification is the gold standard that assures you that a physician is an expert in a specialty or subspecialty. The American Board of Medical Specialties (ABMS) is the medical organization that oversees physician certification by developing standards for the evaluation and certification of physician specialists. To be board-certified, a doctor must complete a residency (post-medical school training) in his or her specialty that has been recognized by ABMS, followed by rigorous written and oral examinations. If a doctor wants to subspecialize, he or she must then complete fellowship training after finishing a residency. For example, to be a board-certified fertility specialist, a medical school graduate must complete a four-year residency in the obstetrics-gynecology specialty, followed by a three-year fellowship in the subspecialty of reproductive endocrinology and infertility.

If that weren't enough, a specialist or subspecialist has to maintain board certification by periodically taking medical courses and passing tests to prove that he or she is up to date. The criteria in each field is specific to the specialty. Some, but not all, board-certified doctors designate their certification as part of their title. For example, a board-certified gynecologist with the letters FACOG after his or her name is a Fellow in the American College of Obstetricians and Gynecologists. ABMS.org is the site where you can check out whether a physician is board-certified and find out what he or she is certified in.

By the way, "anti-aging" is not a specialty recognized by the American Board of Medical Specialties and does not require a residency.

All that is required for certification from the American Board of Anti-aging and Regenerative Medicine is to complete a self-learning course, pass an examination, and submit six patient charts for review by its board. According to its website, only five percent of physicians who have completed this course are gynecologists, which means that ninety-five percent of physicians who practice anti-aging are not experts when it comes to gynecologic exams or treatment of gynecologic issues. It also explains why so many of them prescribe hormones without ever having their patients take off their clothes.

University Affiliations

It's generally a good sign if a physician has an academic appointment at a medical school. Faculty ranks such as instructor, assistant professor, associate professor, and professor depend on a physician's level of involvement in teaching medical students, his or her research, and the number and stature of his or her publications.

If a doctor is not board-certified or has no university affiliation, does this mean he or she is a bad doctor? Of course not! Many non-board-certified physicians are excellent doctors who keep up with advancements in their field and give very good care. Let's face it, though: If you needed brain surgery, would you go to the brain surgeon who's board-certified, teaches at a medical school, and is current in her field? Or would you pick the brain surgeon who finished a residency but failed her boards, took off five years to be an artist, and then returned and has privileges at a hospital that was in such desperate need of a brain surgeon that it didn't require board certification?

By now, I'm sure you get the message.

But vaginal dryness isn't brain surgery. What you need is someone who has an interest in menopause and a knowledge base. Sometimes this expert is a physician, sometimes an internist, sometimes a gynecologist, sometimes a family practice doctor, and sometimes a physician assistant or a nurse practitioner (more on them later). You may be thinking, But I'm seeing an expert! If a gynecologist isn't an expert in this area, who is?

Even in specific fields, doctors have particular areas of interest. A neurologist may be the world's expert on seizure disorders but not know a lot about stroke. Your ob-gyn may have incredible expertise about twin pregnancies and preterm labor, but she may treat women with vaginal atrophy only a few times a year. So how do you know where a doctor's areas of interest lie?

Referral Services

Most hospitals have a physician referral service and will help you find a doctor who is interested in and knowledgeable about your condition. If the hospital you have chosen is well known as a leader in women's health, then that hospital's referral service is usually a great way to find the right doctor. Keep in mind that the people who work in hospital referrals are obligated to make referrals to all the physicians on staff. So if you just call up and say, *"Hi, I have a dry vagina. Which ob-gyn is good?"* you'll most likely be given the name of whoever is next on the list.

You need to ask specific questions that will lead you to the doctor who is most appropriate for you. For example, instead of saying, "I need a gynecologist because sex hurts like hell," you might try, "I'm looking for a board-certified gynecologist who has been in practice for at least five years. I would prefer a woman and would like someone who takes care of a lot of menopausal problems and has identified herself as having an interest or expertise in sexual issues."

You can get a lot of information from a referral service, and it is well worth your time to say exactly what's important to you in a doctor. The referral service will also be able to answer questions about office location and accepted insurance. Many hospitals also have a "physician finder" section on their website where you can type in a condition to find the physicians who list it as an area of expertise.

Hospital referral services are not the same as the commercial referral agencies that operate independently of hospitals. Take it from me, referral agencies that advertise in magazines, the yellow pages, or on TV are not a great source. Participating physicians pay to be part of the service and tell the service what to say. As with any paid advertisement, healthy skepticism is appropriate.

Searching Online for a Doctor

The reason for the increasing popularity of doctor-listing websites is that people are desperate for an easy way to find information about a doctor without actually making an appointment. In our digitally driven society, this seems to be a reasonable desire. After all, wouldn't someone who has already been to that doctor be the best judge of how approachable or knowledgeable he or she is?

Keep in mind that consumer referral lists are no better than asking strangers on the street what they think. Typically, there are no more than a handful of "reviewers" who are rating the doctors. The typical doctor sees thousands of patients a year, and the experience of two or three people is hardly reflective of a typical experience. More important, you have no idea who is writing these reviews or what their agenda is. A glowing review may be from the wife or mother of the doctor. A scathing review may be from a disgruntled patient or employee, or from the wife or mother of the competing doctor in town. It has become common for "online profile management" companies to post positive reviews for businesses and products for a fee.

Even if reviewers' comments accurately reflect their experience, they are usually more about how they were treated at the office than about the skills of the doctor. More than one five-star review has been posted because the doctor was "really friendly," "had a "great staff," and offered free estrogen samples.

Professional Societies

Professional societies such as the American Medical Association or the American College of Obstetricians and Gynecologists are all potential sources of referrals. But to find a menopause expert, your best bet is to head to the North American Menopause Society (NAMS) website, www.menopause.org.

North American Menopause Society

The mission of the North American Menopause Society (NAMS), a nonprofit scientific organization, is to promote the health and quality of life of all women during midlife and beyond through an understanding of menopause and healthy aging. To help meet its mission, NAMS developed a certification exam in 2002. Successful completion of the exam provides a doctor with a three-year credential as a NAMS Certified Menopause Practitioner (NCMP). Menopausal medicine has become increasingly complex, so you are lucky if you find a doctor with this level of commitment and competence.

You can pretty much be guaranteed that a NAMS-certified practitioner has the interest as well as the expertise to evaluate and treat any of your menopausal issues, including the sexual ones. To find a certified menopause practitioner, go to www.menopause.org.

Finding Non-MD Clinicians:
Advanced Practice Nurses and Physician Assistants

So is an MD always the best clinician to help you deal with complex menopause issues? Sometimes a nonphysician is more qualified than many physicians when it comes to diagnosing and treating certain conditions. I am a huge advocate of advanced practice nurses (some are nurse practitioners, and some have other advanced nursing degrees) and physician assistants.

In addition, an advanced practice nurse or physician assistant is likely to spend more time with you than most physicians. I know this firsthand because I utilize invaluable advanced practice nurses and physician assistants at the Northwestern Medicine Center for Sexual Medicine and Menopause.

I made the decision to use the words "doctor" and "gynecologist" when referring to a clinician in this book because I am a gynecologist. Also, it would have been cumbersome to use "doctor and/or advanced practice clinician/physician assistant" throughout the book. To add to the confusion, there are many different degrees that qualify a clinician as an advanced practice nurse.

What If Your Doctor Doesn't Have a Vagina?

Frequently, a new patient will say to me, "I've had the same ob-gyn for twenty years, and I love him, but he's a man, so of course there was no way I could talk to him about this! I want a woman doctor who will understand."

As a physician, I can tell you that I don't need to have personally experienced vaginal atrophy to help my patient with vaginal atrophy any more than I need to experience a urinary tract infection to know how to treat one. The gender (and age!) of your clinician really shouldn't matter. Really.

Obviously, if you are totally uncomfortable being examined by a man or talking to a man about intimate issues, you will be better off with a woman doctor. If you feel somewhat guilty discriminating in this way, consider the number of men who go to women urologists. On the other hand, it would be foolish to go with the less-qualified doctor based solely on gender, so keep an open mind.

Many women go to a woman gynecologist because they subconsciously—or even consciously—think that talking to a female gynecologist will be like talking to a girlfriend. Although it is generally easier to talk to a girlfriend about sex than to your doctor, you are not looking for a new friend at the doctor's office.

You have plenty of people to invite to parties and have lunch with. When choosing your gynecologist, you are looking for someone who has the skills you need and whose judgment you trust. Your doctor need not be your friend, but she or he does need to be someone who will talk to you, listen to you, and help you. Sometimes that person is a woman, and sometimes it's a man.

Mention What You'd Like to Discuss When You Make Your Appointment

When you book an appointment, this is a good time to mention that you have an issue you would like to discuss. You can simply say, "In addition to my annual exam, I have some concerns related to pain during sex." It will then be noted as the reason for your visit, making it more likely that your doctor will bring up the issue. Some women find it easier to mention their concerns to the assistant who brings them into the examination room. The assistant lets the doctor know that the patient has brought up a specific topic, and then the doctor is likely to initiate the conversation.

Make a Separate Appointment

Often a patient will come for her annual "well woman" visit with multiple issues she wants to discuss. When I explain that there is not enough time to deal with all the problems in one visit and that another appointment needs to be made, sometimes I get an unhappy patient. I understand. You've taken time off from work, parked, and paid your copay. An additional visit is not only inconvenient but also expensive. But there simply isn't time to adequately address complex gynecological issues at the time of your annual exam, and they can't—and shouldn't—be quickly tagged onto your routine visit.

Many women are reluctant to make an additional appointment, because their insurance may cover only "well woman" visits and not "problem" visits. But face it, you are having a problem! You deserve and need more time. Your doctor is going to take the time to evaluate and treat the problem if that is specifically why you've made an appointment to see him or her. If it is important enough to you to mention the problem, give yourself permission to go for another appointment. Most initial visits at the Northwestern Medicine Center for Menopause last one hour. Most annual visits for a well woman exam allot fifteen minutes.

Consider Seeing a Menopause Specialist, Even If Your Insurance Doesn't Cover It

Even if you do your homework, you may simply not have access to a menopause expert. You may live in a small

town, or your insurance may keep you locked into a particular group of physicians. Good health care is our right,
and I believe every man and woman should have access to
a doctor who can help them, but sometimes the care you
need is not available within the limitations of your health
care plan. If you really feel that you can't discuss your issues with your current doctor, or if your doctor seems truly clueless or embarrassed when you bring them up, bite
the bullet and spend the money to see someone who can
fix your vagina, even if that person is not covered by your
insurance plan. Keep in mind that it is likely that you will
need only one or two consultations. And you do not need
to end your relationship with your regular gynecologist,
whom you can continue to see for routine visits.

If All Else Fails . . .

If you have a hard time talking to your doctor about your
sexual issues and you don't have the option of seeing another practitioner, I hope that this guide at least helped
you identify your issues and gave you ways to fix them. If
you think you need to see a pelvic physical therapist, ask
your doctor for a referral. If you need a prescription for a
local estrogen, just ask for the one you want. Most likely,
your doctor will just give you the referral and the prescription, no questions asked. You're welcome!

A Word About Sex Therapy

Thanks to the popular HBO series Masters of Sex, pretty much everyone has heard of Masters and Johnson, the
father and mother of sex therapy. And thanks to Masters
of Sex, women who visit the Northwestern Medicine Center for Sexual Medicine and Menopause (the center that
I run) are too often horrified at a referral for sex therapy,
thinking that they are going to be observed having sex

in a laboratory through a one-way window. In fact, contemporary sex therapists do not observe their clients having sex ever! They also do not have sex with their clients, EVER!!!! Sex therapy is talk therapy with both individuals and couples.

Finding a Therapist with Expertise in Sexual Health

I have a staff of sex therapists at my center, but most clinics do not. So if you are not in the Chicago area, your best bet is to find a therapist certified by the American Association of Sexuality Educators, Counselors and Therapists (AASECT.org). AASECT-certified therapists not only have advanced degrees and experience as therapists, but they also have undergone specific training regarding the causes and treatment of low sexual desire, arousal, and orgasm, as well as pain.

In general, sex therapy is short term (approximately three months). Treatment is conducted in an individual, couples, or group setting. Again, sex therapy is talk therapy and may include sexuality education, counseling, and often couples exercises, including sensate focus. AASECT-certified therapists are experts in treating women who have chronic pelvic pain from medical conditions such as endometriosis, a history of sexual trauma, desire discrepancies, or post-menopause sexual problems, just to name a few.

You may have a terrific therapist who helps manage your anxiety and depression but simply doesn't have the training to help with your vaginismus.

Beware the Self-Proclaimed Sex Therapist!

It shouldn't surprise you that there are plenty of people who call themselves sex therapists who have not had the extensive training required to have AASECT certification.

There are two categories of self-proclaimed sex therapists:
- A licensed therapist who has not had formal training in sex therapy but has an interest and has «self-taught» or taken some courses. This is hit or miss. They may do a good job or have no idea what they are doing.
- People who have no professional training and are not even licensed therapists. These folks often call themselves 'sex coaches'. **Steer clear. ▼**

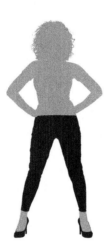

> *FAST-FORWARD: Francey invites her new bestie Linda to go with her to Paris. During walks in the Tuileries Garden and long lunches involving at least two bottles of wine (thanks, Grandma!), they talk for hours about the challenges of getting their post-menopause vaginas in shape. Both grateful to now be able to have pain-free pleasure, they decide that they need to tell all of their friends! Clearly, everyone's dry vagina story is different. Who knew that post-menopausal vaginas could be so complicated? But they are now ready to tell the world that everyone's dry vagina is fixable whether through just a little lube, a lot of laser, rings, creams, or other things.*

13

WRAPPING UP

IT'S CONFUSING. Clearly, there are a lot of tools out there to alleviate vaginal dryness and pain—lubes, moisturizers, local estrogens, DHEA, ospemifene, systemic estrogens, pelvic physical therapy, dilators, lasers. Where to begin?

It really depends on the severity of your issue. There is a huge difference between the woman who says, "It doesn't feel as wet as it used to," and the woman who hasn't had anything even approach her vagina for twenty years because it was so excruciatingly painful the last time she tried. What follows are some general guidelines.

Category 1: On The Dry Side

You are able to have intercourse, and sometimes it's okay, but more often than not, it feels dry and scratchy. Sometimes it really hurts.

Apply a generous amount of lubricant (chapter 4) to the outside of your vagina and all over his penis. If intercourse becomes pain-free and pleasurable, there is no need to do anything else other than have frequent intercourse. And have plenty of lube on hand.

Some women find that even if a lubricant works, they don't want to use one just at the time of intercourse and would rather do something that will keep things wet and ready to go anytime. If that's your preference, try a long-acting vaginal moisturizer (chapter 5), a local vaginal estrogen product (chapter 6), vaginal DHEA (chapter 7), ospemifene (chapter 8), or a laser (chapter 9). You are not required to have severe atrophy to be prescribed one of these solutions.

Category 2: Lube Isn't Doing It

The lube helps, and you are able to have intercourse, but it still hurts.

Despite making things slippery, lube will not be enough if your vaginal tissue is thin and has lost its elasticity. You need to use either a long-acting moisturizer, a medication, or a laser to get the tissues in shape. If you want to try a local estrogen product, DHEA, or ospemifene, you will need to see your doctor to get a prescription. No matter which product you choose, use it for at least fourteen days before you attempt intercourse again.

Also, you need to use a lubricant even if you are using a long-acting moisturizer or prescription product. In one study, forty percent of women discontinued using their local estrogen product because "there wasn't enough relief." Just because you are using estrogen doesn't mean you don't also need a lube.

If things are fine once he is inside, but the entry still feels tight and dry (and if the lubricant doesn't help), use a vaginal estrogen cream at the vestibule of the vagina daily for two weeks, and then taper to one to two times per week.

If intercourse becomes pain-free and pleasurable, great. Do not stop using the moisturizer or prescription product! I guarantee you that things will get dry again if you do. You are not suddenly going to start making estrogen.

After a few months, it is fine to increase the time between doses. If your atrophy is not severe, and, most important, if intercourse occurs on a regular basis, some women are able to use the local vaginal estrogen only once a week or the long-acting moisturizer only once a week. That is great—not because it is safer, but because it is cheaper and more convenient. But if you taper down to once a week and things start to get dry, obviously you need the estrogen and/or moisturizer twice a week, and there is no getting around it.

Category 3: Things Are Bad . . . Really Bad

He can't even get it in there.

And the thought of it terrifies you.

You are going to need to get a prescription for a local vaginal estrogen product, DHEA, or ospemifene or have CO_2 laser treatments. Your vagina is broken and needs to be repaired. Don't panic. Just get a prescription.

Stop trying to have intercourse. Before you have penetration with an actual penis, start pelvic floor physical therapy (chapter 10) or, if not available, home dilator therapy. Once you are successful with dilators, continue to work with them until you are able to get a dilator in that is slightly larger than the penis in your life. When you first attempt to have intercourse, use a generous amount of lubricant, and be in a position that puts you in control if things are not going well. A warm bath beforehand will help relax you and your vagina.

If things are going well, keep using whichever product is keeping your tissues healthy. Twice weekly is recommended for maintenance if you use the cream or tablet, but I have the occasional patient who is dry unless she uses it three times a week. The key is consistency! It doesn't work if you stop using your estrogen for months and then decide to use it on date night.

If you are not making progress with the dilators, you are unable even to get a small dilator in, or you are still having pain, you need to be evaluated by a gynecologist who can check if the tissues are healthy or if there is another issue going on. If everything checks out, you probably have pelvic floor pain and dysfunction from muscle memory and will need pelvic floor physical therapy.

This is fixable!

It is just no longer a do-it-yourself project.

Use It or Lose It

Don't underestimate the importance of having intercourse on a regular basis once vaginal elasticity and pain-free intercourse are restored. "Use it or lose it" is one of those phrases that actually has some truth to it. Regular stimulation of vaginal tissue helps maintain blood flow, which in turn increases lubrication and elasticity. Women who have had a long sexual hiatus are more likely to experience vaginal dryness than women who are regularly having intercourse.

But to be clear, if you are having pain, "use it or lose it" does not apply. It will just make the pain worse. Once your painful vagina is fixed is when "use it or lose it" comes into play.

So what's a woman to do when she's between partners, or has a partner who's out of business, to keep her tissues from drying up?

Regularly inserting a dildo or a vibrator will help maintain vaginal lubrication and elasticity. Many women self-pleasure with vibrators that just provide clitoral stimulation, which works great to have an orgasm, but doesn't stimulate vaginal tissue. A rabbit style vibrator will accomplish both goals. And just like going to the gym, you will enjoy it once you get started!

So if you have no pain but, alas, no partner, stimulate with a device to keep things good to go.

Use it or lose it. ▼

RESOURCES AND TERMINOLOGY

ALTHOUGH I RECOMMEND these resources as containing information that is generally up to date and accurate, my endorsement doesn't mean I agree with everything that appears in these books or on these websites. This section also contains information on some of the over-the-counter products and devices mentioned in the book. No one paid to be mentioned in this book or included in this resources section. This is not meant to be a comprehensive list. Many products that are safe and effective are not included.

MENOPAUSE TERMINOLOGY

Menopause. Menopause is defined as the final menstrual period which is confirmed once someone has not had a period for twelve months. Of course, for women who do not have periods (women who have had a hysterectomy, uterine ablation or use an IUD), this is not a useful benchmark. Essentially, menopause is when the ovaries are no longer producing ovarian hormones, primarily estrogen. The average age of menopause in the United States is 52, but it is normal to enter menopause any time after age 40.

Perimenopause. This is the period of time prior to menopause. Ovarian activity is inconsistent and while some women have no symptoms, other women experience irregular periods, hot flashes, mood swings, and insomnia. This period of time can last months, or years.

Induced menopause. Menopause that occurs as a result of surgical removal of the ovaries, or as a result of cancer treatments such as pelvic radiation or chemotherapy.

Post-menopause. Life after menopause. You are post-menopause until you die.

Premature menopause. Menopause occurs at or before the age of 40. In many cases, this is genetic but may also be the result of an autoimmune disease or induced by surgery, or cancer treatments.

Pre-menopause. Pre-menopause starts with puberty and continues until perimenopause. A fifteen-year-old is considered to be "pre-menopause"

Primary ovarian insufficiency (POI) is defined as when the ovary winds down before the age of 40. It may be permanent, in which case, it is premature menopause, or it may be temporary. POI is often confused with premature menopause. Premature menopause is permanent. In POI, ovarian activity kicks in again.

GENERAL MEDICAL INFORMATION

Check out Chapter 11 (Calling Dr. Google) for additional information about the following recommended websites.

Up To Date
www.uptodate.com
General medical information for physicians and other health care professionals which requires a paid subscription, but there is also a free patient portal.

Mayo Clinic
www.mayohealth.org
This site is good for general medical information about specific symptoms, tests, and procedures.

PubMed
www.ncbi.nlm.nih.gov/pubmed
This site is where medical journal articles are published. Sometimes the full article is available but sometimes it only gives a brief summary and redirects you to the journal website which requires a subscription for full access.

ALTERNATIVE AND COMPLEMENTARY MEDICINE

The National Center for Complementary and Integrative Medicine
www.nccih.nih.gov
Accurate, up- to-date safety and efficacy information on specific herbs, supplements, and practices (such as acupuncture).

FINDING AN EXPERT

The Northwestern Medicine Center for Sexual Medicine and Menopause www.Sexmedmenopause.nm.org
The Northwestern Medicine Center for Sexual Medicine

and Menopause is the center I founded and oversee. Located in Chicago, it is part of Northwestern University and is staffed by experienced physicians, advanced practice nurses and physician assistants. All are certified menopause practitioners of the North American Menopause Society. We work collaboratively with other physicians, certified sex therapists, and pelvic floor physical therapists. We have programs for menopause, vulvar and vaginal health, bone health, and sexual function. It is worth the trip to Chicago.

The North American Menopause Society (NAMS)
www.menopause.org
If you are not in Chicago, the North American Menopause Society's website is the place to go to find a certified menopause practitioner. On the homepage, click on the "For Women" tab at the top, then go to "Find a Menopause Practitioner." Once the list of providers in your ZIP code comes up, be aware that "NCMP" designates a NAMS certified menopause practitioner who has met specific criteria. If someone is not certified, it means they have paid to be a member, and though they are interested enough in menopause to join NAMS, they have not passed the certification exam.

American Board of Medical Specialties (ABMS)
www.abms.org
This organization oversees physician certification by developing standards for the evaluation and certification of physician specialists. Go to the ABMS website to find out whether a physician is board-certified.

Federation of State Medical Boards (FSMB)
www.fsmb.org
Visit this website to verify that a physician is licensed.

SEX THERAPISTS
American Association of Sex Educators,
Counselors, and Therapists
(AASECT) www.aasect.org

PELVIC FLOOR PHYSICAL THERAPY
Pelvic Floor Physical therapists Trained by Herman &
Wallace Pelvic Rehabilitation Institute
www.pelvicrehab.com

American Physical Therapy Association (APTA)
Section on Women's Health
www.aptapelvichealth.org/ptlocator

SEXUAL PAIN AND SEXUAL HEALTH RESOURCES
Sex Rx: Hormones, Health and Your Best Sex Ever,
by Lauren Streicher, MD

*When Sex Hurts: A Woman's Guide to
Banishing Sexual Pain,*
by Andrew Goldstein, Caroline Pukall,
and Irwin Goldstein

Pelvic Pain, Explained,
by Stephanie A. Prendergast and Elizabeth H. Akincilar

International Pelvic Pain Society
www.pelvicpain.org

DOMESTIC VIOLENCE AND SEXUAL ABUSE SUPPORT
Many people experience intimidation, threats, or even
physical harm in their relationships or during contact
with others, whether at home, outside, or at work. Here
are some of the resources available to you regardless of

your gender identity, race, age, citizenship status, or sexual orientation.

National Domestic Violence Hotline
1-800-799-SAFE

National Human Trafficking Hotline
1-888-3737-888 or text *BEFREE to #233733*

Rape, Abuse, and Incest National Network
www.RAINN.org
800-656-HOPE (800-656-4673)
The nation's largest anti-sexual-violence organization has thousands of trained volunteers available 24/7. Please note that if you call 1-800-656-HOPE, a computer will note your area code and the first three digits of your phone number.

RELATIONSHIP BOOKS

Taking Sexy Back, by Alexandra Solomon, PhD

Loving Bravely, by Alexandra Solomon, PhD

Mating in Captivity: Reconciling the Erotic and the Domestic, by Ester Perel, PhD

Love Worth Making, by Stephen Snyder, MD

Come as You Are, by Emily Nagoski, PhD

OVER-THE-COUNTER PRODUCTS

Below are some of the over-the-counter products and devices mentioned in the book. No one paid to be mentioned in this book or included in this resource section.

This is not meant to be a comprehensive list. Many products that are safe and effective are not included.

LONG-ACTING VAGINAL MOISTURIZERS
Replens Long Lasting Vaginal Moisturizer
polycarbophil-based moisturizer
www.replens.com

Revaree hyaluronic acid-based moisturizer
www.hellobonafide.com/products/revaree

Hyalo Gyn Gel hyaluronic acid-based moisturizer
www.hyalogyn.com

LOW OSMOLALITY WATER-BASED LUBRICANTS
World Health Organization:
Full list of osmolality of commercial vaginal lubricants:
 apps.who.int/iris/bitstream/handle/10665/76580/
WHO_RHR_12.33_eng.pdf;jsessionid=849958F8DB-
CD902D1F23041BDE7C6776?sequence=1

Good Clean Love
System Jo
Slippery Stuff
Pulse H2Oh!

SILICONE LUBRICANTS
Replens Silky Smooth
Pulse
Aloe-ahh
Wet Platinum
JO Premium Personal Lubricant
PINK Silicone Lubricant
SLIQUID Organics silk

VULVAR SOOTHING PRODUCTS

Aquaphor Healing Ointment
www.aquaphorus.com

Replens Moisture Restore External Comfort Gel
www.replens.com

Hyalo Gyn Gel
www.hyalogyn.com

TO RESTORE NORMAL VAGINAL PH

RePhresh
www.rephresh.com

Replens Long Lasting Vaginal Moisturizer
www.replens.com

VAGINAL DILATORS

Soul Source
www.soulsource.com

Intimate Rose
www.IntimateRose.com

Milli (a single dilator that expands)
www.milliforher.com

PELVIC FLOOR-STRENGTHENING DEVICE

ATTAIN treats urinary and bowel incontinence. (Full disclosure: I have a financial relationship with this product, which has been clinically proven to reduce both urgency and stress incontinence.)
www.incontrolmedical.com

Acknowledgments

I DECIDED NOT to go the traditional route of publishing *Dr. Streicher's Inside Information Series*. I have been very lucky as an author and have always had a literary agent and a publisher willing to pay me an advance, edit, format and market my books. But, in exchange for those advantages, there is something every author gives up when working with a traditional publishing house. Control. Once the book is sold, it is the publisher's call what the author can, should, and must include.

I admit I am a little bit of a control freak, whether it is in the operating room, or in the kitchen. With Dr. Streicher's Inside Information series, I decided I wanted to do it my way. Even the most talented editor or publisher does not have what I have—thirty years of experience taking care of women, running a menopause clinic, and listening to the concerns of thousands of women from all over the country.

I also would like to emphasize that although many products are recommended in the book, no one paid to be mentioned in this book. When it comes to prescription products, I included every FDA approved option available at the time of publication.

While I do not have an agent or publisher to thank, there are a number of other people who made this series possible.

Thank you to my dear friend Rick Kogan for introducing me to Joe Darrow who is responsible for the fabulous cover design, the Francey image and the overall format. I am honored and grateful that this extraordinary artist, on a ridiculously tight deadline, took on the challenge of a book on vaginal dryness. Check out his website, *joedarrow.com*, to see his iconic magazine covers.

The talented Talisha Bryan, copy editor extraordinaire, who fixed too many typos, and errors to count after I gave her what I considered to be "a ready to go perfect manuscript". For any writer who doesn't think they need a copy editor, you are wrong.

Rachel Zar, my brilliant daughter, is a much better writer than I will ever be. She is also a talented Marital and Family Therapist, and an ASSECT certified sex therapist. I have the pleasure of working with her in the Northwestern Medicine Center for Sexual Medicine and Menopause. Rachel reviewed copy, edited out the bad stuff, and gave me the kind of advice most daughters never have to give their mothers.

I met Suzy Ginsberg years ago when I did a commercial for a tampon that eliminated vaginal odor. The vagina talk and laughter has never stopped. Not only has she become my one woman support group but I count her among my dearest friends.

Lorraine Devon Wilke, a friend and talented author, (check out her books on Amazon!) was a wealth of information regarding the intricacies of publishing.

Francey O.- my childhood friend, who my character is not based on, (other than the smart and witty part) for letting me borrow her name.

I am terrible at social media. I forget to post, I forget

to tag, I forget to link, I still can't figure out Instagram. Forget Tik Tok. It took me awhile to admit it (I am one of those people who has a hard time admitting I am bad at anything) and hire someone who could do it right. So, a huge thank you to Dorothy Hagmajer who not only did not make fun of me for my ineptitude but is making sure that I am "getting out there" on Facebook, Twitter, Instagram, YouTube and LinkedIn. Dorothy, I love that you share my passion for giving women good information that will actually make a difference. And while I am at it, thank you to every single person who follows me on social media and keeps the conversation about menopause alive and relevant.

To Brad Ginsberg and all the folks at Global Communications Works. There are a lot of PR companies. This is a company that not only understands the world of vaginal health, but is also better than anyone else at getting out the word. Thank you!

My patients continue to inform me. It's one thing to make recommendations based on the scientific literature, but it is the real life experiences of the women who use these products that give me the real education.

I am lucky to be part of an amazing group of academic menopause experts. Every year we gather at the North American Menopause Society conference and drink, eat, drink, laugh, drink, and yes, share information about updates in research and clinical practice. All of these folks are my go to sources and collectively know so much more than I will ever know! (Sorry if I forgot anyone!) Risa Kagan, MD, Pauline Maki, PhD, Lisa Larkin, MD, Stephanie Faubian, MD, James Simon, MD, Marla Shapiro MD, Jan

Shifren, MD, Andrew Goldstein,MD, David Portman, MD, Leah Milheiser, MD, Sharon Parrish, MD, Sheryl Kingsberg, PhD, Rebecca Thurston, PhD, Mary Jane Minken, MD, Tara Allman, MD, Diana Bitner, MD, Brian Bernick, MD, Miriam Greene, MD, Nicole Jaff PhD.

A special shout out to my colleagues at The Northwestern Medicine Center for Sexual Medicine and Menopause, Traci Kurtzer, MD, Kristi Tough DeSapri, MD, Rajal Patel, MD, Pat Handler, MSN FPN-C, Sarah Hwang, MD, Audrey Fenwick, MS,PA-C, Rachel Zar, MS,LFMT,CST, Jennifer Levy, MA, LCPC, Shantae Williams, PT,DPT, Toshiko Odaira, PT,DPT and Helene Strange, PT,DPT,OCS. They are all extraordinary clinicians who are responsible for the success of our programs.

To my brothers, Paul, Michael and Ian, and my sisters-in-law Liz and Kim who proudly display my vagina books in their homes, and to our daughters, Rachel, Danielle, Jessie and Julian who I love dearly. I am so lucky to have family that I not only love, but truly like.

And finally, to Jason, my extraordinary husband who had no idea what he was signing up for when he promised to love me "in sickness and in health". In the months before I wrote this book, Jason nursed me through a difficult surgery followed by a life threatening bout with Covid-19 pneumonia. Even if he did not give the best foot massages on earth, he would be the love of my life.

Printed in Great Britain
by Amazon

27772981R00086